CW00408575

QUICK GUIDES

A Healthy Pregnancy

BⱩXTREE

Advice to the Reader

Before following any advice contained in this book, it is recommended that you consult your doctor if you suffer from any health problems or special condition or are in any doubt.

First published in Great Britain in 1995 by Boxtree Limited, Broadwall House, 21 Broadwall, London SE1 9PL

Copyright © Liz Earle 1995
All rights reserved

The right of Liz Earle to be identified as Author of this Work has been asserted by her in accordance with the Copyright, Designs and Patents Act 1988

10 9 8 7 6 5 4 3 2 1

ISBN: 0 7522 1680 5

Text design by Blackjacks
Cover design by Hammond Hammond

Except in the United States of America this book is sold subject to the condition that it shall not, by way of trade or otherwise, be lent, resold, hired out or otherwise circulated without the publisher's prior consent in any form of binding or cover than that in which it is published and without a similar condition including this condition being imposed upon a subsequent purchaser

Printed and Bound in Great Britain by Cox & Wyman Ltd., Reading, Berkshire

A CIP catalogue entry for this book is available from the British Library

Contents

Acknowledgements 4

Introduction 5

1 Preconceptual Care 7

2 The Early Months 19

3 The Middle Months 36

4 Exercise 52

5 The Final Months 57

6 Preparing for the Birth 64

7 The First Few Days 81

Glossary 88

Useful Addresses 90

Further Reading 93

Index 94

ACKNOWLEDGEMENTS

I am grateful to Carla Smith for helping to produce this book. Also to nutritionist Dr Stephen Davies; Dr Ray Rice; aromatherapist Geraldine Howard; herbalist Anne McIntyre; homoeopath Dr Andrew Lockie and acupuncturist Sarah Moon. I am also indebted to the talented team at Boxtree, and to Rosemary Sandberg and Claire Bowles Publicity, for their unfailing enthusiasm and support.

Introduction

Having a baby is a wonderful thing – but it's also a time of great change and uncertainty. We are suddenly surrounded by a whole new world of medical jargon, folklore and other people's well-intentioned advice. Many much larger books have been written on the subject, but this *Quick Guide* aims to cut through the waffle and present you with all the facts you need to know. In addition, I have included specialist advice on a wide range of alternative therapies which can be very useful during pregnancy and childbirth. These include aromatherapy, homoeopathy, acupuncture and herbalism. However, I have not overlooked the very important role of modern medical intervention and the effective forms of drug-based pain relief for childbirth.

As a mother of two small children, I hope I have passed on in this small book some useful tips to help make your own pregnancy the joyful occasion it should be.

Liz Earle

——— 1 ———
Preconceptual Care

Deciding to have a baby is one of the most creative and exciting choices we can make in life. Pregnancy should be a joyous and unforgettable experience which ends with one of the most incredible human miracles – a newborn child. With this new life come new challenges – and the transition to parenthood for you and your partner. If you have decided to try for a baby, it's well worth taking several steps towards good health care for you and your partner before conception. Like many things in life, preparation is everything – especially when it comes to a healthy pregnancy and childbirth.

Although pregnancy isn't like running a marathon, you will find it easier both to get pregnant and to enjoy the nine months of pregnancy with a well-tuned body. Being in good shape will also give your baby the best conditions in which to develop into a healthy human being.

Planning for Parenthood

Getting pregnant is not always as simple as it sounds. You may conceive the first time you try or it could happen several months later. The average woman takes six months to conceive and you may have to wait as long as eighteen months. When planning a baby, it's worth preparing your body from about three to six months before you actually want to conceive. Start to exercise regularly – about three times a week, for twenty minutes each session. Try swimming, jogging, walking, aerobics or playing tennis. This will get your body ready for the load-bearing requirement of pregnancy and the demands of labour. It will also provide a healthy environment in which the foetus can develop.

If you have been taking the contraceptive pill, change to barrier or natural methods of contraception for three months before you want to conceive. This will help your body get back to its normal patterns and prevent any doubts about the time of conception. You may wish to visit your doctor before you conceive – just for a general check-up and for advice on fertility, conception, antenatal care and any other questions you may have on childbirth. It's also worth having a blood test to check that you are immune to German measles (rubella). This illness is mild in adults and children, but can have terrible effects on an unborn child during its first twelve weeks of life. If you are not immune, you should have a vaccination and avoid conceiving for three months.

CONCEPTION

Every month, one of your ovaries releases an ovum, or ripe egg – this is ovulation. The egg travels down your fallopian tube and it is at this point that it may be fertilised by your partner's sperm.

During intercourse, your partner will ejaculate sperm into your vagina. Most sperm leak out of the vagina, but some will swim up through your cervix into your womb and then into your fallopian tube. Conception takes place if a sperm meets an egg and fertilises it. During the week after fertilisation, the egg moves slowly down the fallopian tube and into your womb. It then attaches itself to the thickened womb lining and an embryo begins to develop.

Ovulation usually occurs from twelve to sixteen days before your next period, whatever the length of your cycle (taking day one as the first day of your period). If your periods are fairly regular you can work out which day of the cycle ovulation is likely. Home testing kits are available from chemists which can also tell you when you are ovulating.

As the egg lives for about twelve to twenty-four hours after it has been released from your ovary, you are more likely to conceive if you have sex within this time. Sperm are able to live for several days inside a woman's body, so if you have intercourse a day before ovulation, you are maximising your chances of conception.

MALE FERTILITY

Being prepared about six months before you both want to conceive is not as far-fetched as it sounds. For successful conception, it is as important for the male partner to be in good physical shape as it is for the female, particularly as male sperm take about three months to form in the testes.

To maximise his fertility, a man should:

* Stop smoking
* Stop drinking alcohol or cut back to two–three units a day (no binges!)
* Improve his diet (see Food for Thought below)
* Take nutritional supplements – including zinc – which can increase sperm counts, and a good multivitamin

FEMALE FERTILITY

If you're reading this and are already pregnant, but didn't take any of the recommended steps before conceiving, don't worry. The vast majority of pregnancies do result in a healthy baby, and advice on preconceptual care is just another way of ensuring that those eating an inferior diet can alter their lifestyles before conception.

To maximise her chances of conceiving, a woman should:

* Stop smoking
* Stop drinking
* Improve her diet (see Food for Thought below)
* Take nutritional supplements – including zinc and folic acid (see Essential Extras below)
* Stop taking the contraceptive pill three months in advance
* Stop taking all drugs and medicines unless absolutely necessary

Food for Thought

A healthy diet and lifestyle is vital for you and your partner in the months before conception and in the early stages of pregnancy – to ensure a healthy baby. 'From the preconceptual point of view, if males are boozers and smokers, then the quality of their sperm will be affected,' says Dr Stephen Davies, Director of Biolab, a research unit which studies the role of diet and nutrition in the prevention and management of illness. 'If, in addition to smoking and drinking, the males are on a poor diet, then the effects of those toxins are going to be all the greater ... We live in a twentieth-century polluted environment and the better the diet, the more resistant we are to those toxins and the way in which they detrimentally affect reproduction.'

Focusing on your diet in the months before conception will mean that your bloodstream has the right amount of nutrients needed for the first phase of the baby's growth. Equally, your partner should be eating well to ensure he produces healthy sperm – so maximising your chances of conceiving.

Foresight, the Association for the Promotion of Preconceptual Care, was set up both to help protect the health of unborn children by advising on care before conception and to examine the environmental effects on preconceptual health. The Association recommends that both partners follow a wholefood diet for several months before they try to conceive. This diet can be followed throughout your pregnancy – and is particularly important during the first three months of your baby's development, as this is when the limbs, skeleton and major organs are formed.

The Foresight diet advises you to avoid convenience and processed foods and to eat as much fresh produce as possible. Drinking filtered or bottled mineral water is part of the Foresight plan, which suggests that you and your partner vary your eating habits by choosing and combining from the following four main food groups each day:

Cereals: Eat wholewheat bread, if possible made from organic flour, and wholegrain cereals such as sugar-free muesli. Whole rye, barley, oats, millet, buckwheat, sesame, sunflower seeds and nuts are all good dietary staples.

Dairy products: Whole milk, yoghurt, butter, cheese, eggs and fromage frais are excellent sources of protein and calcium. It's worth choosing the low-fat and semi-skimmed dairy products to avoid a high intake of saturated fats. But soft cheeses and goat and sheep products should be avoided in pregnancy because of the danger of contracting listeria – an infection which can affect the baby and even cause a miscarriage or still birth. For the same reason, make sure you cook any eggs well.

Vegetables, fruits and juices: Eat fresh raw fruit and vegetables as often as possible or have your food very lightly cooked, except for potatoes and unsprouted pulses. Have a fresh salad every day using ingredients such as lettuce, white or red cabbage, cress, cauliflower, radish, tomato, celery, watercress, green and red pepper, carrots and button mushrooms. Liven up your salads with sprouted pulses such as alfalfa and mung beans, or with different kinds of nuts – such as walnut or pine kernels.

Over-boiling or frying vegetables can destroy their valuable vitamin and mineral content. Instead, use a stainless steel vegetable steamer. Shallow rather than deep-fat frying will also maintain more of the vegetables' goodness.

Protein foods: Include all red meat, heart, sweetbreads, tongue, poultry, game and fish (especially shellfish and roe). Buy your meat as fresh as possible and look for organic and free-range varieties. Foresight also recommends that you consider switching to foods such as venison, rabbit, game birds, pigeons and all seafood, as the animals have been in their natural environment and are not intensively farmed. Roast or stew your meat with stock or vegetables – the stock will contain much of the meat's valuable nutrients. Steer clear of liver, kidney, and pâtés – because of the possibility of listeria. Large quantities of liver should also be avoided as they contain high levels of vitamin A, which may be harmful to the foetus.

What to avoid
It's worth cutting out all white flour and white flour products (such as bread, cakes, pasta and white rice) from your pre-pregnancy diet. Sweets, jams and fizzy drinks should also be off your menu as these have very little nutritional value. Never eat potatoes with green patches – these contain a poisonous alkaloid called solanine, which can cause spina bifida in babies. Try to cut out tinned vegetables which are usually high in salt and may contain sugar and artificial colouring. Foresight also recommends that mothers-to-be don't eat tinned meat, commercial

pâtés, bacon, sausages, or packet ham which often contain preservatives and monosodium glutamate.

ESSENTIAL EXTRAS

As well as ensuring you and your partner are eating well, there are various supplements each partner can take to promote a healthy pregnancy.

Folic acid

The most vital vitamin supplement a woman can take before and during the first twelve weeks of her pregnancy is folic acid, a vitamin B supplement. It is essential for the proper development of the neural tube (which becomes the baby's spine) – this takes place in the first four weeks of pregnancy. If the spinal vertebrae do not fuse properly, the baby can be born with spina bifida, which affects nearly 2,000 pregnancies each year.

Neural tube defects are preventable by taking folic acid before pregnancy and during the early weeks. Unfortunately, by the time most women realise they are pregnant it is too late, as the neural tube will have already closed over. For this reason, there is a move to fortify all breads and cereals with folic acid (some already are – check the package).

Folic acid is available naturally in green vegetables, but a pregnant woman's diet usually contains only one-third of the amount needed to prevent a baby's handicap.

You can buy folic acid supplements in all good chemists. The Government has recommended that pregnant women take a supplement containing 0.4mg of the vitamin a day – before and up to the twelfth week of their pregnancy. Dr Nicholas Ward of St Bartholomew's Hospital suggests that a supplement is taken for at least a few weeks prior to pregnancy, and for the first five weeks of pregnancy. St Bartholomew's Hospital operate a Helpline (see Useful Addresses) to give guidance on folic acid.

The message is, if you are thinking of getting pregnant, or if there is any chance that you might become pregnant, take a folic acid supplement to protect the child's health.

The zinc link

Zinc can play a vital part both in conception and a healthy pregnancy. This mineral is essential for the growth of most living things – especially babies! Low levels of zinc have been found in stillborn babies and in men with fertility problems. Fertility problems and lack of sex drive in women have been linked to a lack of zinc, and a deficiency of the mineral during pregnancy can lead to restricted foetal growth. Mothers who are low in zinc can have more complications during the birth. Zinc is found in all meat and fish and is present in plant seeds such as sesame and sunflower seeds, wheat and oat germ and sprouted seeds such as alfalfa. But, to be extra sure of a sufficient zinc intake, you and your partner should start taking a zinc supplement a few months before you intend to conceive. A good daily intake is from 15 to 20mg (make sure you take the elemental as opposed to the compound zinc). You'll double your absorption of the mineral if you take it with vitamin B6; but try to avoid drinking coffee after taking zinc – this can halve the amount you'll actually absorb.

Smokescreen

If either you or your partner smoke it could hinder your chances of conceiving. Smoking reduces the levels of vitamin C in the body and a study by Professor Bruce Ames of the University of California has found a clear link between low levels of this vitamin and genetically damaged sperm. Smoking damages DNA by oxidation and so causes genetic damage that could be inherited. Professor Ames warns that men who smoke and eat a nutritionally inadequate diet are risking damage to their sperm, 'an effect that will reverberate down the generations'. Professor Ames' study also found that 'paternal smoking appears to increase the risk of birth defects and childhood cancer in offspring'.

Female smokers are also damaging their chances of having a child. Maternal smoking can cause problems such as slow development of the foetus in the uterus leading to spontaneous abortion, premature birth and low infant birth weight. A report from the Royal College of Physicians, *Health or Smoking*, concluded that, 'Women who smoke are more likely to be infertile or take longer to conceive than women who do not smoke.' The Royal College of Physicians found that over 4,000 miscarriages of healthy foetuses occur because of maternal smoking during pregnancy. In its report, *Smoking and the Young*, the Royal College concluded that maternal smoking during pregnancy and infancy is 'the most important avoidable risk factor for infant death'.

Smoking when you're pregnant can harm the unborn child. Carbon monoxide passes from your cigarette through your lungs into your bloodstream, and prevents your baby receiving as much oxygen as it should. As a result, the baby won't grow as well as it should. Having a smaller baby does not make childbirth any easier (the head stays roughly the same size), and the child will be weaker. It goes without saying that giving up the nicotine habit can only be beneficial if you're planning to have a baby. But if you find it impossible, try to cut down on cigarettes, or visit a hypnotherapist to help you stop.

Think Before You Drink

Having the occasional alcoholic drink is a wonderful way to relax – but is it a good idea if you're planning a baby? Medical opinion varies on how safe it is for pregnant women to drink. A heavy intake of alcohol (eight glasses of wine a day or the equivalent) has been shown to affect fertility and can damage the unborn child.

Babies born to heavy drinkers may suffer from 'foetal alcohol syndrome' (FAS). The children have various facial features in common – including a receding forehead and chin – and suffer from various behavioural and developmental problems as they grow older. About 10 percent of babies born to alcohol drinkers have been found to show some signs of the syndrome.

While some doctors advise that you cut out alcohol completely while you are pregnant, others say that 'moderate' drinking is safe for the unborn baby. Moderate drinking is usually described as one or two alcoholic units once or twice a week. Drinking wine is thought to be less harmful than beer, because the latter contains thiocyanate – also found in tobacco. It is probably better to stop drinking altogether a few months before you plan to conceive, but if you can't, limit yourself to a maximum of two to three units a week before and during your pregnancy.

Toxoplasmosis

This is an infection caused by a parasite which isn't usually dangerous to healthy children and adults but can seriously affect the health of an unborn baby. The parasite, which can't be seen by the naked eye, is found in raw meat, cat faeces and the soil where cats defecate. If a woman catches toxoplasmosis during pregnancy, there's a high risk that it may affect her unborn child. The baby can develop serious symptoms such as water on the brain (hydrocephalus), brain damage which can result in mental handicap and epilepsy, and damage to the retina at the back of the eye causing partial loss of sight or blindness. The baby may not always contract the infection – and most of those who do won't be severely debilitated but eye problems will develop later in life.

Three out of ten people have had toxoplasmosis by the age of thirty, without realising. Some people experience mild 'flu-like symptoms when they have the infection. Once you've had toxoplasmosis, you are immune for life – so it's worth having a test, to find out if you've had it, before you begin to try for a baby. If you are already pregnant, you can be tested at your antenatal clinic. But make sure you understand the implications of the test result. This will be either that you have never had toxoplasmosis and should take relevant precautions; that you have already had the infection and are now immune; or that you have the infection and need further tests and treatment.

The Toxoplasmosis Trust, founded to bring the disease to the public's attention, says that if the infection is caught early in pregnancy, it is less likely to cross the placenta to the baby; but if it does, the effects on the foetus are serious. If, however, the woman catches the infection later in pregnancy, it is more likely to cross the placenta, but won't have such severe effects on the baby. On average, 40 percent of affected mothers pass the disease onto their babies and, of these, 10 percent are likely to be seriously affected by toxoplasmosis.

AVOIDING TOXOPLASMOSIS
To avoid getting the infection:

* Only eat meat which has been cooked through thoroughly – so it's brown with no trace of blood or pinkness.
* Wash fruit and vegetables thoroughly to remove all traces of soil.
* Wash your hands and all cooking utensils and surfaces after preparing raw meat.

* Avoid unpasteurised goat's milk and unpasteurised goat's milk products.
* Wear rubber gloves when gardening and wash your hands afterwards.
* If your child has a sandbox, cover it to prevent cats from using it as a litter tray.
* Delegate someone else to change the cat's litter tray.

—— 2 ——
The Early Months

The first part of your pregnancy, or first trimester, runs from when you became pregnant to about fourteen weeks. This is a crucial time for the growing foetus, as its major organs and spinal cord are formed. So it is vital for you to eat well, rest and take excellent care of your newly pregnant body.

After conception (most likely about two weeks after the first day of your last period) the fertilised egg travels into your womb, where it attaches itself to the lining. When the egg is firmly attached, conception is complete. At this point, the embryo (as it is now called) extends tiny finger-like projections called villi. These push into the lining of the womb to reach your blood-stream, from where they obtain nutrients for the growing embryo. The villi will later mature to form the placenta, which provides all the nourishment the foetus needs until birth (see Glossary). Some of the embryo's cells start to form the baby's organs and from weeks three to four the neural tube begins to develop. This will become the baby's brain and spinal cord.

By the end of the fifth week, the embryo is 1cm ($3/8$") long and is floating in a fluid-filled sac. It now has a simple brain, spine and central nervous system and its heart has begun to beat. Blood vessels link it to the placenta via the umbilical cord.

From weeks six to eight the embryo undergoes a dramatic development. Its arms and legs become clearly visible, bone cells begin to develop and all the major internal organs develop in simple form. By week eight the embryo, now called a foetus which means 'young one', is 2.5cm (1") long – about the size of a strawberry.

During weeks nine and ten, the embryo's eyelids begin to form, it has recognisable fingers and toes and its genitals begin to develop into male or female. By the end of week ten, the fundamental parts and internal organs are fully developed.

From weeks eleven to twelve, the foetus' body has grown so the head no longer seems so large. His or her eyes, ears and tooth roots have formed and he or she will have skin and nails. At twelve weeks your baby begins to move around – but you won't be able to feel it yet!

By the fourteenth week the foetus is recognisably human, with a definite profile. Some of its major organs have formed and its movements are now more active and coordinated. It can move its head and lips and has swallowing and breathing reflexes. It now measures 8–9cm (3³/₄") long.

How Do You Feel?

While all this activity is going on in your womb, you may be experiencing a variety of physical changes. During the first part of pregnancy you may begin to notice changes in your appetite and a sudden, inexplicable dislike of some foods and craving for others. Many women become more emotional and sensitive during this period. You may feel nauseous and even vomit at times of the day when your blood sugar level is low, such as early morning and evening.

To combat morning sickness, try eating a dry biscuit or other light snack before you get out of bed. Eat small amounts throughout the day, ensuring you never go for too long without food – many experts believe that pregnancy nausea is related to a low blood glucose concentration.

During the second month you may begin to get out of breath more easily (for example, when climbing the stairs) and may need to pass water more frequently. You may also feel very tired and need more rest than usual – so early nights are an excellent idea.

What Should You Eat?

You may have gone off many foods you liked before pregnancy, but it's important that you continue to eat well during this first stage of your baby's growth. Your baby depends on what you eat and drink for its nourishment in the womb. If you haven't already established a healthy diet, with a little careful planning you can ensure you're eating the right foods and getting enough of the essential vitamins and minerals. Try to eat plenty of fresh fruit and vegetables – a salad a day will certainly keep you and your baby topped up with many of the essential nutrients. And, to boost your energy levels and avoid that common pregnancy niggle – constipation – eat a diet rich in unrefined carbohydrates and fibre, such as potatoes, whole-wheat bread and pasta.

Cut back on junk foods and sweet snacks – these have little or no nutritional value and will simply help you to pile on the pounds! If you must eat something sweet, have some fresh fruit such as white grapes to stop the craving. Fatty foods such as chips, cakes and ice-creams are another pregnancy pitfall. Again, try and drop these in favour of healthier foods. To see if you're getting enough of the essential nutrients, check out the box below.

ESSENTIAL PREGNANCY DIET

Protein: Women who aren't pregnant are recommended to eat about 1½oz (46g) of protein each day. You may need twice as much during pregnancy, as it is needed for the growth and repair of cells both in your body and the baby's. Protein is found in fish, meat, nuts, pulses and dairy foods. Animal sources of protein can be high in fat, so try to limit your consumption of these.

Carbohydrates: You need these for energy and to help the body to use protein efficiently. They are found in sugar and in many types of food you may eat as part of your everyday diet, such as bread, flour, cereals and potatoes.

Fats: Fats are a major source of energy and help the body function normally. Before and after pregnancy your fat intake should be less than one-third of your diet. Good sources of fat can be found in oils such as sunflower and olive, nuts and seeds, and dairy products.

Calcium: You need about twice as much calcium as normal during pregnancy. The Recommended Daily Allowance (RDA) for calcium for pregnant women is 1,200mg a day – up about 400mg from the RDA for non-pregnant women. As your baby's teeth begin to develop very early in pregnancy, your calcium intake during the first four months is important. It is found in cheese, milk, yoghurt, leafy green vegetables, whole grains, pulses and nuts.

Vitamin C: Very important as it helps to build a strong placenta, helps your body fight infection and promotes iron absorption. Found in fresh fruit and vegetables, such as oranges, grapefruit, strawberries, broccoli, potatoes and cabbage.

Folic acid: You need twice as much of this vitamin as normal during pregnancy. It is essential for the development of the baby's central nervous system in the first few weeks of pregnancy (see page 13). Found in fresh green leafy vegetables such as broccoli, as well as chick peas, soya beans, wheatgerm and lentils, but take a supplement to be on the safe side.

Iron: Your body will need increased amounts of iron during pregnancy as iron is a vital ingredient of haemoglobin, the substance that carries oxygen to your baby via your bloodstream. Around one-third of your iron intake is used by the baby to create blood and build up its own stores. It is found in red meat, green vegetables and dried fruit. If your iron count is low, your doctor will give you an iron supplement to boost your intake.

Zinc: This mineral helps in healthy growth and brain and nerve formation (see page 14). It may also prevent morning sickness. It is found in beef, liver, seafood, nuts, carrots, bananas, tomatoes and wholegrains, or take a good elemental zinc supplement. Drinking coffee and alcohol may inhibit your absorption of zinc. Taking zinc supplements is also a good idea over the nine months as some research has suggested that a lack of zinc during pregnancy can lead to smaller babies and a longer labour. One London study found that women with small babies had significantly lower concentrations of zinc in their white blood cells.

Vitamin B12: If you're a vegetarian and worried about getting enough of the right nutrients, it's well worth taking a vitamin B12 supplement. This vitamin helps to form haemoglobin and the baby's central nervous system. It is found in meat, fish, poultry, wholegrain cereals and dairy products.

CUT BACK ON CAFFEINE

You may see your daily cups of tea or coffee as one of life's essentials, but it is a good idea to cut back on these during pregnancy. Both drinks contain caffeine, an addictive stimulant which can over-activate the nervous system. Drinking coffee or tea can cause the heartbeat to speed up and could have a similar effect on your baby as caffeine (and other drugs) can cross the placenta.

Drinking coffee and tea with or after meals can also prevent you from absorbing vital vitamins and minerals. For example, if you drink tea during a meal, you're reducing your absorption of iron, and if you drink coffee after a meal you can halve the amount of zinc you've taken in from your food. There are many alternatives to caffeine – such as one of the delicious herbal teas currently available. Some are actually good for you and may help with minor ailments – for example, camomile tea is excellent if you are having problems sleeping, and peppermint tea is said to help digestion. Dandelion and chicory coffees are also a useful alternative.

FISH OIL FACTS

A regular intake of fish oil may benefit you and your baby during your pregnancy. The best source of this oil is in dark fish such as herring and mackerel, but if you don't like fish, you can take fish oil supplements.

Fish oil contains substances which are not found in any other oil. All edible oils are made up of fatty acids, but these fall into different categories. Those in fish are called the Omega-3 group of polyunsaturates, which include two very important substances – EPA (eicosapentaenoic acid) and DHA (docosahexaenoic acid). The Omega-3 polyunsaturates have been shown to reduce the tendency of blood to clot, reducing the risk of thrombosis. They also reduce blood pressure and improve kidney function.

Dr Ray Rice, Chief Executive of the Fish Foundation – an organisation promoting the benefits of fish and fish oil – says that fish oil can benefit your pregnancy in three ways.

Prevention of pre-eclampsia

This is a problem which usually becomes apparent in the later stages of pregnancy. The symptoms of pre-eclampsia include raised blood pressure, large weight gain, swollen hands, feet and/or ankles and traces of protein in your urine. Pre-eclampsia (sometimes also called pregnancy-induced hypertension, or PIH) is potentially dangerous to the unborn child as well as to the mother. If allowed to proceed untreated it can, in extreme cases, result in death. It is thought to arise from improper development of the placenta, decreasing the flow of blood through the umbilical blood vessels. This has the effect of reducing the amount of food and oxygen available to the foetus. There is an increased risk of prematurity in cases of pre-eclampsia.

But eating more oil-rich fish (or taking a fish oil supplement) can help to reduce the likelihood of this happening. 'Lack of fish oil is not only a cause of pre-eclampsia,' says Dr Ray Rice, 'But there is evidence to show that if fish oil is present in the diet, the risk of pre-eclampsia is reduced.' Fish oil can reduce the symptoms of pre-eclampsia, such as high blood pressure, and it can reduce the risks of blood clots forming where they are not wanted.

Prolonging the pregnancy

Research has shown that if you have a reasonable amount of Omega-3 in your diet, your baby's gestation period is increased by two to four days. This may sound minimal, but towards the end of pregnancy any extra time in the womb means the baby puts on more weight – ensuring it has fewer development problems in later life.

Helping the premature baby

'It looks as if premature babies have an absolute need for pre-formed Omega-3 polyunsaturates, which you can only get from fish,' says Dr Rice, 'because they can't convert the short-chain derivatives, present in ordinary food, unlike the rest of us and full-term babies.' DHA, a substance found only in fish oil, is vital for a baby's development because 60 percent of the polyunsaturates in the human brain is composed of DHA. 'It is the single most important polyunsaturate in the brain,' declares Dr Rice. And, as the major development in a baby's brain happens during the last three months of pregnancy, clearly it is vital for premature babies to receive an equally good supply of DHA.

'We do know that there's a need for the foetus to have a good supply of DHA in order to develop to its fullest extent and we suspect this is why some premature babies have problems at school. It's quite conceivable that their brain structure is in some way affected by the absence of the short supply of DHA in their last few months in the womb,' says Dr Rice. However, if a premature baby is breastfed, he or she won't suffer any problems, as a mother's milk contains pre-formed DHA – unlike modern formula feeds. To make sure you're getting enough fish oil in your diet, eat dark fish such as salmon, pilchard, kipper or mackerel once or twice a week. If you can't face this, try a fish oil supplement (not cod liver oil, which contains high levels of vitamin A – see page 12). Vegetarians can either forego their principles for a few months or take a linseed oil supplement This contains similar essential fatty acids (although not as effective) as fish oils. Alternatively, buy whole linseed from your health food shop to sprinkle on salad or breakfast cereal.

Body Beautiful

Stretch marks are a problem everyone associates with pregnancy. They may appear over your tummy, breasts and buttocks as dark or reddish streaks, a sign that the skin has been stretched from underneath. After the birth they fade to become a silvery colour. Who gets stretch marks is largely a question of luck and genetics. They are more common in fair-skinned and overweight women. But, by using oils or creams to rub into your skin you may avoid getting them or reduce their potential extent. There are some commercial stretch mark creams available, but you can actually use any oil or cream which is easily absorbed into your skin. Try a daily massage using almond or vitamin E oil or one of the rich vitamin E creams available. While this should help, you may not be able to avoid the odd one or two stretch marks. If you want to avoid stretch marks a good diet is also important as it helps to build strong skin from within. Some nutritionists believe that zinc deficiency plays a part in the development of stretch marks as zinc promotes normal growth and development. It is interesting to note that adolescents and pregnant women need more zinc than everyone else and they are also more prone to developing stretch marks. Vitamins C and E are also essential nutrients for building strong, healthy skin; vitamin C is particularly good as it actually helps to form collagen in connective tissue and so helps to maintain the skin's elasticity, making it less susceptible to developing stretch marks.

Natural Help

Pregnancy affects every woman differently. Your baby's development may hardly affect you physically (until it starts kicking!) or you may experience some of the typical nine-month niggles such as nausea, constipation and extreme tiredness (for solutions see the Natural Pregnancy Remedy Finder in Chapter 3).

As well as the physical side-effects of pregnancy, you might experience wild mood swings about your new state. Perhaps you feel you're not as sexually attractive to your partner as usual, or you worry about putting on huge amounts of weight. You may be concerned about becoming a parent or about the birth itself. Many women are anxious for the unborn child – and fear that it may not be in perfect health. All these concerns and worries are perfectly normal and can be allayed by talking to your doctor or midwife, or to friends who have already had children.

If you are feeling anxious and tired in the first stages of pregnancy, this is the ideal time to learn how to relax and enjoy your new physical condition. Using safe natural therapies such as aromatherapy, flower remedies, homoeopathy or herbalism may clear up your minor physical problems and help you rest and relax.

AROMATHERAPY

This soothing treatment, popular for thousands of years, uses fragrant and powerful essential oils, extracted from flowers, trees and herbs, to treat a wide range of physical and mental problems. Treatment of the whole human being – body, mind and mood – is very important as the physical body and the mind's psyche are closely linked. As well as being used for medical problems, aromatherapy is also useful to promote general health and well-being. It can also help you overcome some of pregnancy's side-effects such as stretch marks, nausea and fatigue.

Aromatherapy works in two different ways – through your sense of smell and via absorption into the skin. Our sense of smell has a profound and immediate effect on the way we feel – probably because smells access the brain directly, particularly the part of the brain dealing with the emotions. Essential oils are easily absorbed by the skin because of their small molecular structure. They are quickly absorbed into the bloodstream and then travel through the entire body via the intricate network of blood vessels, which means they can work on the whole body.

During your pregnancy, you may wish to visit a qualified aromatherapist for a massage, or use some of the essential oils at home for your bath, a burner or massage. Essential oils are too highly concentrated to be used neat on the skin – so, if you're making up your own massage oil, they should be mixed with a carrier or base oil. The most common base oils include almond, avocado, grapeseed and hazelnut. There are some essential oils which should not be used in pregnancy, as they may cross the placental barrier and could, in theory, affect your baby (see below). To be on the safe side, concentrations of essential oils used should be less than for when you are not pregnant.

When making up your own massage oils with a base oil, follow these measurements: 5ml equals 1 teaspoon; 10ml equals one dessertspoon and 15ml equals one tablespoon.

Essential oils to avoid during pregnancy: basil, bay, cedarwood, fennel, marjoram, myrrh, sage.

Essential oils you should use with caution: black pepper, coriander, cypress, ginger and rosemary.

Oils recommended by aromatherapists in pregnancy: citrus oils (tangerine, grapefruit), geranium, lavender, neroli, patchouli, sandalwood, rose, rosewood.

FLOWER POWER

The Bach Flower Remedies, formulated by Edward Bach, a Welsh doctor, are another soothing source of treatment during pregnancy. These thirty-eight different essences contain parts of different wild flowers or plants and work on the principle that if you are feeling bad, this negative state of mind may be expressed as a physical illness. By treating your mind, you can restore health to your body. The remedies are grouped to deal with negative states of mind, including despair, uncertainty, loneliness, fear and tenseness, among others. Thus you could take Wild Rose if you are feeling apathetic or Larch if you are lacking in confidence and fear failure.

The remedies are all available as tinctures – although Rescue Remedy is available in both liquid and cream form – and can be found in most health food shops. The flower essences used in the remedies should be taken diluted in water, but may be used neat in an emergency (such as Rescue Remedy). All are harmless and can be taken during your pregnancy. Just put four drops in a glass of water and sip slowly, or use the glass dropper to put a few drops on your tongue or behind your ears.

Rescue Remedy is one of the better known Bach Flower remedies. This is a mixture of five different remedies – Clematis for bemusement, Rock Rose for terror, Star of Bethlehem for shock, Impatiens for tension and Cherry Plum for desperation. Not only can it be used to deal with shock and faintness during pregnancy, it can help women in labour and immediately afterwards.

HOMOEOPATHIC HELP

Homoeopathy could help you with some of pregnancy's more common physical niggles such as constipation and nausea. This natural medicine was devised in 1790, by Samuel Hahnemann, a German doctor. Unlike conventional medicine, homoeopathy sees physical symptoms as attempts by your body to expel disease. Thus a homoeopath will treat an illness by giving the patient a minute dose of the same ailment – instead of prescribing a medicine to suppress the symptoms. For example, if you had bad diarrhoea, a homoeopath might give you a minute dose of a substance which would cause diarrhoea in a healthy individual. This makes the body fight back and use its own ability to heal.

A visit to a homoeopath begins with a long assessment, with the practitioner asking you all about your emotional and physical history. This is because homoeopaths believe people react differently to the same disease. If you have specific problems during your pregnancy, such as constipation or morning sickness, you can try treating yourself with homoeopathic remedies, but if this fails to work quickly, visit a homoeopathic doctor who can give you the right treatment.

Homoeopathic remedies are available in most health food shops and chemists and come in the form of a soft pill or powder. If you are treating yourself at home with homoeopathy, make sure you follow these guidelines:

* Find a remedy which matches your personality and lifestyle – not just your symptoms.
* Avoid coffee and peppermint (including toothpaste) immediately before or after taking homoeopathic remedies as they lessen the effectiveness of the treatment.
* Dosage: homoeopathic remedies come in different doses. The 6c, 12c and 30c are all safe to take at home. But don't go over 30c.
* Repeat the dosage according to the severity of your symptoms – every ten minutes if you are feeling terrible – and take the remedy less often if there is a distinct improvement.
* If you've taken six doses and there's no improvement, change the remedy, or visit your homoeopath.

HERBAL HELP

One of the oldest natural therapies, herbalism has been used by many generations of women to ease both pregnancy ailments and childbirth. But herbs continue to have an important role to play in pregnancy, and can help you to ease problems such as morning sickness and heartburn.

Herbalism is still a vital part of modern healing, with traditional plant remedies providing about 85 percent of the world's medicines. Yet, unlike modern drugs, herbs support the healing processes of your body rather than attacking the disease directly. Like homoeopathy, herbal treatment takes all aspects of your lifestyle into account. This includes your past and present medical history, your social, domestic and working environments, relationships, beliefs and emotional state, as well as your diet and your relaxation and exercise routines. While you can treat yourself at home (as long as you know the herb is safe to take during pregnancy), it's also a good idea to visit a herbalist who can properly assess your case.

If you wish to treat yourself with the recommended herbs for pregnancy, you can buy some of the more common herbs in health food shops and use them fresh or dried to make infusions or decoctions. For rarer herbs, visit a specialist herbalist or buy them via mail-order (see useful Addresses). But always stick to recommended dosages (refer to the Natural Pregnancy Remedy Finder in Chapter 3).

Most herbs can be drunk in an infusion or decoction which can be made like a tea.

* Infusions are made using the soft parts of the herb such as leaves and flowers. For an infusion, use one or two teaspoons of the herb in a cupful of boiling water, or one ounce of the herb to one pint of water.

* Decoctions are made by using pieces of wood, bark or root, broken into tiny pieces or powdered. For a decoction, put the herb in a pan covered in the same amount of water as above, plus a little more to make up for any lost in the process. Then leave it to simmer for five to ten minutes.

If you're using fresh herbs, twice the amount of the herb should be used in teas – because of the extra water content of the plant. You can generally drink three cups of your herbal remedy each day for chronic conditions and six for acute conditions.

Herbs to avoid during pregnancy: arbor vitae, autumn crocus, barberry, black cohosh, bloodroot, blue cohosh, broom, cotton root, feverfew, golden seal, greater celandine, juniper, life root, male fern, mistletoe, mugwort, nutmeg, pennyroyal, poke root, rue, sage, southernwood, tansy, thuja, wormwood.

Herbal teas recommended for pregnancy: Red raspberry leaves. Recommended by doctors and midwives for many generations, these can help the digestion and the nerves. But most importantly, they are said to normalise the function of the muscles of the uterus – and so help to ease the birth. Start drinking raspberry leaf tea once or twice a day when you are six months' pregnant; eight weeks before your due date, increase this to two or three times a day.

Camomile tea. Helps induce sleep.

Peppermint tea. A good digestive.

Nettle tea. Rich in iron and a good pregnancy tonic. Helps to ease leg cramps.

Problems in Pregnancy

Sadly, not all pregnancies are problem-free or go the full term. Miscarriages are fairly common in the first three months of pregnancy, and usually happen because there is something wrong with the baby. About one in six pregnancies end in miscarriage. The first sign that you may be miscarrying is usually vaginal bleeding. However, this may only be a threatened miscarriage and so will not result in the end of your pregnancy. It could be a suppressed period – which happens when there is not enough pregnancy hormone to stop your period. If this is the case, the bleeding will eventually stop and the pregnancy will continue as normal.

Early miscarriage is quite like a period, with bleeding and similar aching pains, which may occur around the time that a period is due. If you begin to bleed, contact your antenatal carer immediately. You may be advised to get some bed rest or go to the hospital as quickly as possible. If the bleeding continues and the baby's heartbeat cannot be picked up by ultrasound scan, the miscarriage is inevitable and there is virtually nothing that can prevent it from happening. But if the ultrasound does pick up the baby's heartbeat, there is only a small chance that you will miscarry, even if the bleeding continues for a while.

It is three times as rare to miscarry after the twelfth week of pregnancy as it is for it to happen before this time. Bleeding and labour-type pains are the signs of a late miscarriage. After a miscarriage, you may be given a 'D and C' or a dilation and curettage, to empty the womb. This is done under general anaesthetic.

Many women feel a strong sense of loss and sometimes even guilt after having a miscarriage. Although a miscarriage can happen at any time, it is easy to fool yourself that a row, love-making or a late night may have caused it. However, the truth is that a miscarriage is rarely somebody's fault. If you do miscarry, allow yourself to grieve for the lost baby and talk about the way you feel to your partner and close friends or family.

One miscarriage will not affect your chances of conception – and even after three miscarriages you still have a good chance of a normal pregnancy. But if you do have three or more, you should ask your doctor for a thorough examination, blood tests and ultrasound scans.

PLACENTA PRAEVIA

Bleeding in the second half of pregnancy may be caused by placenta praevia – when the placenta is planted too low in the uterus. This condition can happen in four different grades. The first grade is when only part of the placenta lies in the lower area of the uterus. The fourth grade is more problematic and the placenta is completely in the lower part of the uterus and lies over the cervical canal.

Vaginal bleeding without any pain is an indication of placenta praevia. Bleeding may have been brought on by intercourse or straining. Placenta praevia can be confirmed by an ultrasound scan which will establish the position of the placenta. If you have the condition, you will probably be made to rest in bed in hospital until the foetus is mature – up to the 37th or 38th week of pregnancy. If you have third or fourth grade placenta praevia, it is very likely that your baby will be induced at 37 or 38 weeks, before labour begins.

ECTOPIC PREGNANCY

In a normal pregnancy, the egg moves down the fallopian tube to the womb to develop. But sometimes it attaches itself to the tube and grows there. If you have missed a period and are suffering from severe pain in your lower abdomen, vaginal bleeding, and faintness or dizziness, visit your doctor immediately, in case you have an ectopic pregnancy.

An ultrasound scan can diagnose an ectopic pregnancy, and an abdominal operation is necessary to remove the egg. If the fallopian tube is very damaged, it may also have to be removed.

3

The Middle Months

You may find the mid-term stage (fifteen to twenty-eight weeks) the most enjoyable part of your pregnancy. Your body has adapted to its new state and you will probably be over the early nausea and tiredness. More exciting is the fact that you are now actually beginning to look pregnant with your bump gradually growing larger.

Many women feel very well during this stage and begin to bloom as their skin and hair reaches excellent condition. It's also an ideal time to make the most of your new-found energy and start regular exercise such as swimming or yoga.

What's Happening to the Baby?

Your baby is fully formed by the sixteenth week and, during the second trimester, he or she grows rapidly; by week twenty-eight the baby will weigh about 900g (2lb).

During the fourth month (weeks sixteen to twenty), the baby's eyebrows and eyelashes grow and also a covering of fine downy hair (called lanugo) to maintain the correct body temperature. Baby will grow to 14cm (5½") from head to bottom and will weigh nearly 0.25kg (½lb).

You may feel the baby's first movements in the fifth month (weeks twenty to twenty-four), if you haven't done so already. Some women describe this as a faint fluttering in their womb or a slight bubbling feeling. Your baby will probably begin to react to external noises at this time by kicking gently.

In the sixth month (weeks twenty-four to twenty-eight), your baby's sweat glands form under the skin and the arm and leg muscles will be well-developed. The eyelids, previously glued shut, open at around the end of this month or the beginning of the seventh. You will now feel kicking and punching movements as the baby moves inside you. You may feel coughing and hiccuping as a tiny knocking movement! The baby can now hear and recognise your voice and may show appreciation of certain types of music by his or her movements. A baby born at the end of the twenty-sixth week has a chance of survival with the help of intensive care.

By the twenty-eighth week, your baby is beginning to develop fat under the skin and can now feel pain and responds in much the same way as a full-term baby.

Your Body

You will probably feel the urge to eat more than usual, and may be tempted to stuff down sweet and non-nutritious foods. Try to stick to a wholefood diet and the healthy eating and living guidelines described in Chapter 2. During the second and third trimester you should eat about 300 kilocalories a day above your normal intake of food. From the fourth month, a weight gain of one pound a week should be all you're putting on – with an overall pregnancy weight gain of twenty to thirty pounds.

Many women worry that they are putting on too much weight during pregnancy – but much of the weight is linked to the baby. You must take into account the weight of the baby, the placenta, the amniotic fluid, the increase in volume of your blood and your enlarged uterus and breasts. One good way of assessing if you're putting on too much weight is to measure your upper thighs each week and keep a record of any changes.

This will show any increase in your own body fat, as opposed to weight gained from the pregnancy.

Never diet during pregnancy as you and the baby will begin to miss out on vital nutrients. At the same time, try not to put on too much weight as this will put extra stress on your muscles and ligaments and make it harder to assess the baby's development.

Natural Pregnancy Remedy Finder

During the middle stages of pregnancy you may find you begin to suffer from minor ailments such as heartburn and constipation. But you can easily help yourself by using a natural therapy such as homoeopathy, herbalism or aromatherapy, or by making simple changes to your diet and lifestyle. Common ailments with natural remedies and self-help tips are listed alphabetically.

ANAEMIA
If you find you're suffering from exhaustion, fainting and breathlessness, you may be anaemic. When you're pregnant, your blood is supplying your baby's placenta with oxygen, as well as your own body. The amount of blood in your body increases from about seven pints (four litres) to nine pints (five litres) by the end of your pregnancy. But the haemoglobin (iron) content remains constant – which means it will drop by about 20 percent in each pint of blood. If you're worried you may be anaemic ask your doctor for a blood test. Symptoms of anaemia are pallor, white fingernails, tiredness, weakness and fainting.

Herbalism:
Some herbs, such as nettle, raspberry leaves, gentian, hawthorn and vervain, contain iron. These can be used in teas. You can

also add leafy herbs to salads or cook them as a vegetable. Try dandelion leaves and rocket for added flavour in salads.

Homoeopathy:

Use Ferrum metallicum (if you're pale and exhausted), or alternate this with Calcarea phosphoricum – these should help your body to absorb iron more effectively.

Helping yourself:

Eat more iron-rich foods such as plenty of green vegetables (cabbage, broccoli), eggs and wholewheat products. Anaemia caused by a lack of folic acid can be rectified by eating lots of green, leafy vegetables and taking folic acid supplements. Anaemia caused by lack of vitamin B12 (common in vegetarians) can be cured by eating foods which are rich in this vitamin such as brewer's yeast (Marmite contains yeast extract), seaweeds and algae. Iron tablets containing extra vitamin C or tissue salts which aid absorption and assimilation can be taken by those who lack iron. Try cooking with iron pans, as small quantities of the metal dissolve into your food. Floradix is an excellent herbal iron tonic available from health food shops. Unlike conventional iron pills, it does not cause constipation. However, if you are not anaemic, it is neither necessary nor advisable to take iron supplements during pregnancy.

BACK PAIN

Low backache is very common in pregnancy. You are using different muscles in your lower back from those you would use when not carrying a baby and this often leads to muscle strain – particularly uncomfortable during the third trimester. Another reason for your low back pain may be the pressure of your baby on the nerve roots in this region, which can result in painful muscle spasms. Thirdly, your pregnancy hormones have a relaxing effect on the ligaments binding your pelvic joints together, which allows them to expand to provide more room for the growing baby. But the relaxation of these ligaments can affect your spine and this, combined with the growing weight of your uterus, means you get backache.

Aromatherapy:
Ask your partner to massage your back with 50ml almond oil, and ten drops of a mixture of any of the following essential oils: citrus, geranium, patchouli and sandalwood.

Herbalism:
For muscular tension, try drinking relaxing teas such as camomile, lemon balm and skullcap. For muscle pain, try massaging with a few drops of lavender and rosemary or ylang-ylang essential oil, mixed in 50ml of a base oil.

Homoeopathy:
If your back feels weak and tired with dragging pains in the middle and lower back, take kali carbonicum. Belladonna should be taken if your head feels hot and there is a hard, tense feeling in your lower abdomen. If you have this hard tense feeling and feel hot all over, take Pulsatilla. If you feel chilly and also have this hard, tense feeling in the lower abdomen, take Nux vomica. Other remedies to choose from are Arnica, Bryonia, Hypericum and Rhus toxicodendron.

Helping yourself:
Slouching puts more strain on your lower back, so try to stand taller and avoid leaning on one leg – stand firmly on both. Avoid wearing high heels and make sure you're sleeping on a good mattress. When sleeping, try lying on one side with a pillow behind your back and one between your legs – this will relieve pressure on your spine. Daily exercise will also help to

tone and strengthen your muscles. See the Back Strengthener exercise in Chapter 4.

COMMON COLD

You may catch more colds during pregnancy, because hormonal changes can cause the mucous membranes of the nose and sinus to swell. As a result, colds and coughs can be harder to clear up than usual.

Aromatherapy:

Put two drops of eucalyptus, lavender and lemon into a bowl of almost boiling water. Inhale the steam for ten minutes.

Herbalism:

Take half a teaspoon of echinacea in a little water every two hours. This is available in a tincture from most chemists. Or drink an infusion of catmint or ginger tea three or four times a day.

Homoeopathy:

Take Aconite. Don't use nasal drops or inhalants when using homoeopathic treatments.

Helping yourself:

Your body may be telling you to slow down so get some rest and early nights. Drink lots of fluids and eat plenty of fruit and vegetables, avoiding dairy products and junk food. Taking a zinc supplement, garlic capsules and extra vitamin C may help.

CONSTIPATION

Very common in pregnancy as food moves at a slower rate through the intestines, due to the relaxing effect of your pregnancy hormones which decrease the muscle tone of the bowels. Your growing uterus also takes up more space, previously occupied by most of your intestines. As your intestines are compressed, your digestive system slows down even more. Constipation can also be caused by taking an iron supplement.

Aromatherapy:
Massage your back, outer buttocks and thighs with 50ml of almond oil containing ten drops of rosewood essential oil, eight drops of melissa or neroli and eight drops of patchouli.

Herbalism:
Some herbs can be made into teas to stimulate the bowels, without irritation – linseeds and psyllium seeds, yellow dock root, orange peel, camomile and dandelion root.

Homoeopathy:
If your constipation is accompanied by a dull headache and a feeling of fullness in the rectum, then take Nux vomica and stop as soon as it improves the problem. For hard, dry, burnt-looking stools accompanied by a thirst for large quantities of fluid at infrequent intervals, take Bryonia. If you produce large, hard stools and experience shooting pains in the rectum, take Sepia. Alternatively, if you have no desire to pass stools unless the rectum is full and find it difficult to pass even soft stools, take Alumina. If you never empty your bowel properly and have difficulty passing hard, small stools and are also passing a lot of wind, take Lycopodium.

Helping yourself:
Make sure you're eating plenty of fibre – from fruit, vegetables and wholegrains (apart from wheat). Try to cut out bread and wheat products for a while as they can have a blocking effect, and eliminate dairy products and meat as they also block up your gut. Drink lots of fluids, avoid using laxatives and try

taking vitamin C supplements (3–5g per day). Try drinking hot water or tea with lemon as soon as you wake up, and then wait half an hour before you eat or drink anything else. This may stimulate your bowels. A few spoonfuls of linseeds taken with a large glass or two of water is an excellent day-to-day regulator.

CRAMP

You may experience this in your calves during the night, when the muscles are tired. It is a common complaint during pregnancy, and may be caused by circulation changes or calcium deficiency.

Aromatherapy:

Massage with 30ml almond oil containing two drops of citrus oils or geranium oil.

Herbalism:

Make a tea from a herb high in calcium such as horsetail, nettle, comfrey, kelp or meadowsweet. To help poor circulation make ginger root or hawthorn leaf tea. To relax muscular tension, try a decoction made from cramp bark.

Homoeopathy:

For cramp which is worst in the calves and which is relieved by warmth and walking, take Veratum viride. If the cramp in your calves and soles of the feet is accompanied by numbness or pins and needles in the arms and hands which is worse in cold weather, take Nux vomica. For cramp which mainly afflicts the left leg and which wears off once pressure is applied, take Colocynth, and for legs which feel cold and numb, take Ledum. Another good homoeopathic cure for cramp is made by dissolving tablets of the tissue salt Magnesium phosphorica in a glass of warm water and drinking it when you feel the cramp starting.

Helping yourself:
When the cramp starts, massage and stretch the muscle by extending your heel and pulling your toes towards you. Eat more calcium-rich foods, or take a calcium/magnesium supplement – the problem could be related to a mineral imbalance. Regular exercise should also help. See also the Calf Stretch exercise in Chapter 4, and the Leg Massage in Chapter 5.

CYSTITIS
This inflammation of the bladder, and other urinary tract infections, occurs in pregnancy because the bladder and kidneys are working harder to deal with increased body fluid and the pressure of the uterus.

Aromatherapy:
Soak in a warm bath or sitz bath (just a few inches of water) with four drops of bergamot and two drops of lavender or six drops of tea tree oil.

Herbalism:
Alternate drinking plenty of water or barley water every twenty minutes with cups of herbal tea made from any of the following: marshmallow, horsetail, camomile, corn silk or raspberry leaves.

Homoeopathy:
There are a number of different remedies you can take. At the first sign of discomfort, especially if the weather is cold and windy and you feel feverish and restless, take Aconite. If you leak urine at the slightest tension, take Pulsatilla. If your bladder and urethra feel itchy and irritable and if you pass dribbles of urine frequently and with difficulty, take Nux vomica.

Helping yourself:
Flush out your kidneys by drinking plenty of water – try having a glass every half-hour if it's particularly bad. Drink cranberry juice, as it helps prevent E coli (the organism responsible for most urinary infections and diarrhoea) from sticking to the cells of the bladder and urethra. Eat an alkaline diet, with lots of fruit, vegetables and whole grains. Keep yourself warm and put your feet up.

EXHAUSTION/FATIGUE

You will probably feel very tired in early pregnancy, more energetic in the middle months and need plenty of rest in the last trimester. But continuous tiredness is unusual and may be connected to anaemia or anxiety.

Aromatherapy:
Soak in a warm bath with one drop of mandarin, one drop of reviving ylang-ylang and two drops of rosewood oil.

Herbalism:
In later pregnancy, rosemary tea is very good – or try vervain and wild oats as teas or tinctures. For anxiety take skullcap, vervain and camomile tea and, for exhaustion, try cinnamon.

Homoeopathy:
If you feel mentally exhausted, take Anacardium; for headaches and general exhaustion from overwork, take Silica. Alternating tissue salts Kali phosphorica and Calcarea phosphoricum can be of great help for nervous exhaustion.

Helping yourself:
Get as much rest as you feel you need and eat a well-balanced diet. Try to keep up some form of gentle exercise such as yoga or swimming. Supplement your diet with an organic multivitamin and mineral tonic and a B vitamin complex.

INDIGESTION AND HEARTBURN

You may find that some foods give you indigestion during pregnancy – tea, coffee and spicy foods are often responsible. Heartburn, an unpleasant burning sensation in the chest, is caused when the muscle between the oesophagus and stomach relaxes in later pregnancy. The enlarged uterus forces acid upwards from the stomach and causes the heartburn.

Aromatherapy:

Use 10ml of almond oil with two drops of sandalwood, or two drops of orange or mandarin essential oil to massage your solar plexus – the area between your breasts and your bump.

Herbalism:

Make a tea from meadowsweet – and drink at least two to four cupfuls in sips during the day. You could also use marshmallow, peppermint, camomile, lemon balm, fennel, liquorice or dandelion root.

Homoeopathy:

Take Nux vomica to begin with, but if this does not prevent indigestion and you also experience bloating and flatulence, then take China. If fatty foods are responsible for your indigestion and you are also vomiting and suffering from lack of thirst, take Pulsatilla.

Helping yourself:

Eat smaller more frequent meals and eat slowly so plenty of saliva is released, helping the food to digest partially before it reaches your stomach. Avoid any foods that you know make the problem worse, such as spicy food, bread, dairy products, sugar or meat. Eating alkaline foods which can neutralise the acid, such as yoghurt and milk, will help ease the problem. Ask your pharmacist for a remedy containing the mineral magnesium which effectively neutralises the acidity. Make sure it is a formulation safe to take during pregnancy.

INSOMNIA

As your pregnancy progresses, you may find it harder to get comfortable at night – and be unable to sleep. Your baby's movements may also prevent you from sleeping well.

Aromatherapy:

Put a couple of drops of neroli or sandalwood essential oil on your pillow.

Herbalism:

For a gentle relaxant, try a tea made from either one or a mixture of the following: skullcap, lady's slipper, catnip, lime-flower or vervain. Also calming are camomile, lemon balm and raspberry leaves.

Homoeopathy:

If your insomnia is caused by over-excitement and over-stimulation of the mind, take Coffea. To abolish the feeling that you will never get to sleep again, especially as the result of some form of grief, take Ignatia. Take Aconite if your insomnia is accompanied by a feeling of fear. As a general remedy, try tissue salt Kali phosphoricum once a night for a month before you go to bed.

Helping yourself:

Avoid caffeinated drinks such as tea or coffee and stick to herbal infusions, particularly camomile tea. Try taking a calcium and magnesium supplement before you go to bed. Make sure your bedroom is well-ventilated and your mattress not too hard or too soft. Have a warm, relaxing bath shortly before you go to bed.

MORNING SICKNESS/NAUSEA

Many women experience this in the first three or four months of pregnancy, but some suffer for the entire nine months. Various factors are thought to cause nausea including low blood sugar, low blood pressure, hormonal changes or even ambivalence about being pregnant.

Aromatherapy:

Place a drop of peppermint oil on a handkerchief and inhale.

Herbalism:

Ginger is an excellent remedy. Take up to 1g of the powdered herb in a capsule or take two to five drops of the tincture in water or under the tongue. Drinking ginger beer or eating ginger biscuits is also said to help! Or make a soothing tea from lemon balm, camomile, wild yam, raspberry leaves or peppermint and fennel and sip during the day.

Homoeopathy:

Take Nux vomica if you are vomiting small amounts of food with mucus. For non-stop nausea where everything is vomited up, including liquids, take Ipecacuanha. If you have nausea in the evenings which tends to wear off before bedtime, take Pulsatilla. For sudden vomiting a few hours after eating, take Ferrum phosphoricum and, if your vomit is full of milky mucus and you feel irritable and weepy, take Sepia. If you experience heartburn and are having to eat continuously in order to keep sickness at bay, take Petroleum. For diarrhoea and a burning sensation in the abdomen take Arsenicum album. If you have an aversion to bread, fat and slippery foods, crave salt and feel very thirsty, take Natrum muriaticum. If you're feeling very bad, take Ipecacuanha, but stop as soon as the symptoms improve.

Helping yourself:
Get out of bed slowly and have a drink with a dry biscuit or piece of toast on waking. Instead of tea or coffee, drink a glass of hot lemon and honey or a cup of herbal tea. Eat small amounts about six times a day. If you've lost your appetite, take vitamin B6 as a supplement.

OEDEMA

Some pregnant women experience puffiness in their feet, ankles and hands, which usually disappears after a night's sleep. It is thought to be caused by gravitational pull combined with the increase in body fluids and fluid retention. Occasionally, puffy ankles can be a sign of high blood pressure.

Aromatherapy:
Use 50ml of almond oil and ten to twelve drops of lavender or citrus oils – massage your legs with this every day.

Herbalism:
Drink raspberry leaf tea, or a gentle diuretic such as cornsilk, dandelion leaves, camomile, meadowsweet or couch grass.

Homoeopathy:
A short course of Natrum muriaticum may help mild swelling. If your swelling is accompanied by chilliness and restlessness, take Arsenicum album, and for swelling which is accompanied by inflammation and stinging pains that are made worse by heat and slight pressure, take Apis mellifica.

Helping yourself:
Rest as much as you can and exercise regularly to create healthy muscle tone. Take brewer's yeast supplements (as long as you are not intolerant to yeast). Rest your legs up against a wall or armchair as often as possible.

VARICOSE VEINS

Small veins in your legs may swell up, become painful and show during pregnancy. This is because the volume of blood increases when you're pregnant, which stretches the walls and the valves in the veins. This can cause blood to gather in the lower limbs – resulting in varicose veins.

Aromatherapy:

Never massage directly over varicose veins, but stroke the oil into the skin above the vein. Use 50ml of almond oil with ten drops of geranium, eight drops of cypress and four drops of peppermint.

Herbalism:

Herbal lotions can be made to bathe the problem area. You can make up a basic lotion of one part witch hazel (available from any chemist), one part glycerol and three parts water. Or steep some marigold (calendula) flowers in a cupful of distilled witch hazel for an hour and apply with cotton wool or a flannel. Alternatively drink a tea made from hawthorn, limeflowers, shepherd's purse or St John's Wort.

Homoeopathy:

As a first resort take Pulsatilla; if this does not work and the skin is marked with knotted, painful veins, take Carbo vegetabilis. If one foot is hot and the other is cold, take Lycopodium. If you are in pain, take Hamamelis.

Helping yourself:

Try to avoid standing for long periods and exercise regularly to maintain your muscle tone. Splash your legs with cold water – this will help alleviate the soreness of inflamed veins. Make sure you sit with your feet up for a short time each day. Support tights are also very useful, but need to be put on in the morning before you stand up – so keep a pair beside the bed and wriggle into them! See also the Leg Massage in Chapter 5.

—4—

Exercise

While pregnancy is not the time to embark on a strenuous or adventurous new sport such as sky or scuba diving, it is worth maintaining some regular form of gentle exercise during the nine months. If you are already quite fit, you will find exercise during pregnancy easier; if you've done no exercise before your pregnancy, you can always take up a gentle exercise such as regular walking or yoga.

Why exercise during pregnancy? You will feel better – exercise helps your circulation and digestion and helps to stimulate your mind. Regular exercise will also help you to prepare yourself for the birth by strengthening and toning your muscles. Staying fit will help prevent you from putting on too much weight, and may give you more energy – believe it or not, exercise can make you feel less tired! You may also avoid getting some of the typical pregnancy problems such as varicose veins, oedema and cramp. You will also find it easier to relax and will almost definitely sleep better as a result of regular physical activity.

Good aerobic exercise to take includes walking and swimming. Try walking briskly three times each week for fifteen to thirty minutes. Swim gentle lengths at your local pool – any stroke is fine. If you've enjoyed cycling or tennis before your pregnancy then keep it up – but it's not a particularly good time to start these from scratch. Yoga is an excellent activity to take up at this time, as it can teach you useful stretching and breathing exercises which may prove invaluable during the birth. It will also help to relieve stress and allow your body to become more supple. Regular yoga will also help you after the birth – when you want to get back into shape.

Exercising Through Pregnancy

HOW TO EXERCISE SAFELY DURING PREGNANCY

* Never overdo things. If you begin to feel tired, dizzy or strained – stop immediately.
* Warm up properly before you begin and give yourself a chance to cool down and wind down afterwards.
* Make sure you don't overheat – it's not good for you or the baby.
* Don't get dehydrated – drink as much water as you need, before and after.

TIMETABLE
First trimester:
You may feel very tired during the first twelve weeks, so don't exercise too vigorously – stop as soon as you feel tired or strained. It's worth avoiding very strenuous exercises – especially if you have a history of miscarriage.

Second trimester:
You will probably feel more energetic than in the first few weeks, so take advantage of this and take gentle exercise two or three times a week.

Third trimester:
As the birth draws closer you will probably begin to feel tired and heavy. Don't over-exert yourself, but try to continue some form of gentle exercise – it'll make you feel more relaxed and give you more energy.

SIMPLE PREGNANCY EXERCISES

There are several simple stretching exercises you can do at home to tone up your body – some of which involve positions which may help in your labour. These are taught at many pregnancy yoga classes and antenatal groups up and down the country, and are easy to learn and do.

Pelvic floor exercises

A vital exercise – not just for birth, but for life! The pelvic floor is a very important group of muscles, yet many women know very little about them. These muscles lie at the bottom of the pelvis, supporting the womb, bladder and bowels, rather like a hammock. The pelvic floor is shaped rather like a figure of eight – a large loop controls the urethra and vagina and a smaller ring at the back, controls the anal sphincter. These two rings overlap in the centre, the perineum.

If your pelvic floor weakens, you can suffer from a minor leak of urine each time you cough, laugh, sneeze or run for the bus. During birth these muscles are particularly important, as the pelvic floor has to relax and stretch to allow the baby to pass through the vaginal opening.

After the birth, the pelvic floor may weaken, so it's well worth exercising these muscles during pregnancy. To find out where your pelvic floor actually is, try stopping yourself next time you are urinating. Just stop mid-stream and hold briefly, then empty your bladder. It's the muscles you use to stop the flow that you should be using in pelvic floor exercises.

When you've established where the muscles are, try doing this simple exercise every day. Choose a position you feel comfortable in – it may be lying on your back with your knees up, or just sitting on a chair. Now slowly pull yourself in and tighten up from around the back passage through to the middle and then the front. Try to hold for four to five counts and then let go. Aim to do five to ten at first and then gradually build up until you are doing about fifty each day. You can do this exercise anywhere, any time!

Tailor sitting

This exercise helps your pelvic area by improving circulation and widening the pelvic canal, which increases flexibility and relaxes the muscles of your pelvic floor.

Sit on the floor with a straight back, bringing the soles of your feet together. If you need support, sit with your lower back against a wall. Lower your knees towards the floor and breathe deeply. Each time you breathe out, allow your hip joints to relax, so your knees drop further to the floor.

Squatting

This opens your pelvis, strengthens your legs and is a useful position for labour. Stand with your feet 45cm (18") apart. If you want more balance, place your hands against a wall. Lower yourself into a squat, keeping your heels down, if you can.

If you find it difficult to squat, try practising with a partner. Hold on to your partner's arms just below the elbows and slowly lower yourself down, with your knees as far out as possible. Hold for as long as is comfortable, then come up slowly.

Calf stretch

This is an excellent exercise to do if you're getting cramp in your legs. Stand facing a wall, with your palms against it. Step towards the wall with your right leg, keeping it bent, while stretching your left leg, heel flat on the floor. Repeat with the other leg. Do several times.

Pelvic tilt

This helps you to move your pelvis more easily – good preparation for the birth. It will also strengthen your stomach muscles and your back muscles. First, kneel on the floor on hands and knees, making sure your back is flat. Then pull in your stomach muscles, tighten your buttock muscles and tilt your pelvis forwards. Breathe out at the same time. This should make your back hump. Stay in this position for a few seconds, then breathe in and release. Repeat several times.

Back strengthener

If you're suffering from lower backache, this exercise may help relieve it, while strengthening your thighs. Lie on your back with knees bent and feet slightly apart, and with your arms by your sides. Breathing in, tighten your buttocks and lift up your pelvis, pressing down on your heels. Your back should lift off the floor up to your shoulder blades. Remain in this position for a second, then curl down slowly as you breathe out. Repeat several times.

Note: If you feel uncomfortable or faint lying on your back, don't do this exercise.

——5——
The Final Months

You're now approaching the big birth day! During the last three months – from week twenty-eight to the birth – you and the baby will gradually be growing larger, as the baby puts on weight.

By twenty-eight weeks, your baby's eyelids are open and will have eyelashes. He or she measures about 38cm (14") long and weighs about 900g (2lb). The lungs haven't yet matured and need to develop a substance called surfactant, which stops them collapsing between each breath. You may be able to see the shape of a foot or a bottom as the baby moves inside you.

During the third trimester, your baby lays down fat stores and the skin, which was rather wrinkled, now fills out. By week thirty-two, the baby is completely formed, with the body in proportion, 42cm (16") long and weighing around 1,800g (4lb). He or she may also have turned head down, ready for birth, although some babies don't turn until the last week, and about 10 percent do not turn (these are called breech births). From now on, the baby's weight will probably increase by about 200g (7oz) each week.

By week thirty-seven, the baby is larger (so the rolling movements in your womb are less frequent), weighing about 2,250g (5lb) and measuring about 46cm (18") long.

By week forty, the long awaited birth day is near. Most of the baby's lanugo hair will have disappeared; he or she may still be covered in vernix (a creamy-white moisturising substance) or just have a little left in skin folds. The average baby is 51cm (20") and 3,400g (7½lb) at birth.

How Do You Feel?

During the last three months you will look noticeably pregnant, as your bump grows by about ¼cm each week! You should also be able to feel the baby moving around quite strongly – particularly in the first part of this last trimester. Towards the end, as the baby becomes bigger, these movements are less frequent.

You may also begin to feel quite tired – partly due to the extra weight of your baby, placenta, amniotic fluid and enlarged uterus. Your sleep patterns may be broken because you need to visit the loo more in the middle of the night (because of the pressure of the baby on the bladder), and the baby's kicks may wake you up.

Remember to continue following the guidelines on lifestyle and nutrition described in Chapter 2.

By week thirty-two, your uterus will almost fill your abdomen and reach just below your ribs. You might start to experience practice contractions (called Braxton Hicks contractions), which aren't usually painful. This is the uterus preparing itself for labour, but don't worry if you don't feel them as not all women have these contractions.

During the last month, when the baby has turned downwards and the head has engaged in your pelvis, you may feel some relief as breathing may be easier; heartburn and indigestion should decrease, although you'll still be making frequent trips to the loo. But, by the very end of your pregnancy, you'll probably feel rather ungainly, with a heavy feeling in your lower abdomen. It's vital that you relax during your last few days, although you may experience a strong nesting instinct and want to rush around preparing your home for the new arrival. It's very important to rest and relax during the last three months of your pregnancy.

Massage

One way of relaxing any tired or over-stressed muscles is to have a massage. You can either visit a qualified masseur, or ask your partner to treat you with some basic massage techniques. But check with your doctor before you begin.

HOW TO GIVE A PREGNANCY MASSAGE

To give a really relaxing and soothing massage, find a quiet place where your partner can lie on a pile of cushions and – this is optional – a bottle of your favourite aromatic massage oil, perhaps 50ml of almond oil with five drops each of sandalwood, grapefruit and rose or rosewood essential oils.

When massaging a pregnant woman, you should ensure that all your movements are smooth and gentle, rather than applying a great deal of pressure. It doesn't matter that you're not a professional masseur – just use any soft movement that relaxes your partner.

Massage dos and don'ts

* Don't massage anyone under three months' pregnant, because of the risk of miscarriage.
* Don't use heavy pressure on the abdomen and lower back.
* Don't press on varicose veins.
* Don't allow her to lie on her stomach.
* Do keep your movements gentle.
* Do massage areas where there always seems to be tension.
* Do always massage towards the heart.
* Do give a massage just before your partner goes to bed. Ask her to leave the oils to soak into her skin overnight, bathing in the morning.

Useful massage areas

If you're using oil to massage, rub your hands together to warm them up, and then apply the oil to the area you are about to massage. Sit or kneel beside her and begin to work gently on her skin. Tension is often held in the muscles of the lower back, neck and shoulders; a gentle massage can really help to ease the stress in these areas.

Back and shoulder massage

Your partner can either lie on her side on the edge of a bed or sit backwards on a chair, supported by cushions. Using the pregnancy massage oil, push your hands gently along either side of her spine and over her shoulder blades. Then bring your hands down the side of her body. Massage her waist gently with circular movements to help soothe any overstretched ligaments.

Neck and arm massage

Get your partner to kneel comfortably, and place yourself behind her. With fingers of both hands, gently massage the muscles of her neck and shoulders. Then, using the whole of each hand, knead her shoulders. Gradually proceed down her upper arms, massaging the muscles as you go, then massage her lower arms and hands.

Body massage

Gentle strokes on a pregnant woman's abdomen can be very soothing. Place towels on any part of the body which isn't being massaged to keep her warm. The only action on the abdomen should be a gentle clockwise rubbing movement, or stroking.

Leg massage

This can help to alleviate cramp and varicose veins. It also helps to reduce fluid retention. Your partner can sit or lie on pillows. Glide your hands from the ankles up to the thighs and down to the ankles again.

Foot massage

Ask your partner to stay in the same position as for the leg massage. Hold her foot in your lap and use your other hand to stroke her foot from ankle to toes. Work over the whole foot allowing it to bend and flex in your hands. Use your thumbs to massage the sole of the foot, then hold her toes in one hand and gently move them up and down.

Note: Avoid vigorous massaging of the heel, ankle bones and Achilles' tendon – reflexologists believe these to be related to the uterus, and intensive massage may bring on contractions.

Rest and Relaxation

Learning to relax properly is really valuable in helping you overcome any tenseness or minor physical niggles during the last few months of pregnancy. If you attend an antenatal or yoga class, you may learn some very useful relaxation techniques – or you can try this simple method at home.

Either lie on the floor, using pillows to make you more comfortable, or rest in your favourite chair. Close your eyes, and begin to tense and release each part of the body. Start with your face – pull your muscles around, making grimacing expressions, scrunch up your eyes and stick out your tongue. Then slowly relax all your face muscles, including your jaw and tongue.

Next, move on to tense up your neck muscles and relax. Hunch up your shoulders tightly and relax. Tense each arm separately and relax. Tense your abdomen, waist and rib cage and let go. Then move down to your thighs and buttocks, tensing up the muscles and releasing. Next tense your shins, calves and ankles and let go. Then your feet and toes – tighten your toes and flex your feet, then relax.

As you are tensing and relaxing every part in your body, try to switch off your mind and feel your body growing heavier and sinking into the floor. Allow yourself to drift off, forgetting your everyday cares and worries, perhaps imagining yourself on an exotic beach or scenic mountain peak.

After about ten minutes you should be feeling far more mellow and relaxed. This is something you can do several times a week – or whenever you need to slow down.

Another way of helping yourself relax is simply to take a warm, soothing bath. Use one of your favourite essential oils in the water (such as a couple of drops of ylang-ylang or tangerine), and light the room by candlelight, to make it an even more sensual experience. Playing soft music can also help you to wind down in the bath.

Breastfeeding Preparation

If you're intending to breastfeed your baby, the last trimester is a good time to prepare your nipples for the experience. This could help you avoid some of the soreness you are likely to experience in the early days of breastfeeding.

Try to avoid using soap on your nipples as this can have a drying effect, which may encourage cracked nipples later. After you've had a bath or shower, rub each nipple gently with a towel. Then hold the nipple, slowly pull it out and gently, turn it up and then down. Do this several times with each nipple, but don't let it become a painful experience! You can also increase the number of these nipple pulls each time. You may find that this stimulation produces a yellow liquid discharge. Don't panic – this is simply the extra-nutritious colostrum ready and waiting for your baby's first few days.

Some expectant mothers use a skin cream or oil to lubricate their nipples, but any gentle moisturising cream or safflower oil will soften up your nipples. Going bra-less for a small part of each day is also good for nipples, which can benefit from a bit of fresh air and the friction of rubbing against your clothes. It may sound bizarre, but you can also prepare for the experience of breastfeeding by buffing nipples gently with a clean, dry toothbrush.

—— 6 ——
Preparing for the Birth

In the remaining weeks before the birth, it's an excellent idea to prepare your labour bag – so you're not rushing around the house trying to find things at the last minute. Unless you're planning a home birth, you'll need most of the items below.

* A couple of nightdresses (front-opening if you're going to breastfeed) or long T-shirts
* Lightweight dressing gown and slippers
* Two or three nursing bras (or normal bras if you will not be breastfeeding)
* Breast pads to mop up leakages
* Your sponge bag with toothbrush, hairbrush and any other essentials
* Towels
* Two packets of extra-absorbent sanitary pads
* Several pairs of old pants or disposable paper pants (the most comfortable ones come from the National Childbirth Trust mail-order service – see Useful Addresses – and are well worth buying)
* Loose clothes for afterwards
* Change for the hospital pay-phone, and your phone book
* A book or magazines
* Juice or mineral water
* Your favourite cassettes – some hospitals now have stereos in the delivery rooms

* Natural remedies or essential oils which may be useful in labour
* Pure vegetable oil for massage
* Arnica 30c tablets to take after the delivery
* Calendula nipple cream to assist with breastfeeding
* This *Quick Guide* to read while in the first stages of labour and after the birth, so that you have all the information on remedies close at hand

Basics for the baby
* Vests
* A couple of all-in-one baby suits
* Nappies (newborn size)
* Shawl or blanket
* Tissues and cotton wool

Natural Remedy Labour Kits

There are various natural remedies you can take into the delivery room or have by your bed at home, to help ease your labour day.

BACH FLOWER LABOUR KIT
Bach Flower Rescue Remedy may be of great help. Just put a few drops in a glass of water to keep near you in the delivery room, and sip whenever you need a little extra natural help.

HOMOEOPATHIC LABOUR KIT
If you want to take a homoeopathic labour kit to hospital, choose from the remedies listed overleaf (refer to the dosage instructions in Chapter 3).

During birth

Arnica: You can take this throughout labour to prevent bruising. Take every four hours if it's giving you effective pain relief.

Gelsemium: Use if you're drowsy, trembling and shaking.

Natrum muriaticum: Good for relieving backache during labour.

Pulsatilla: Can be used during labour if you're feeling insecure, weepy and exhausted with ineffective contractions.

After the birth

Arnica: Helps to heal bruised muscles.

Calendula: Often used to soothe nipples which are tender after breast-feeding.

Hypericum: Helps heal cuts and stitches (dilute a few drops of tincture in warm water to bathe the area).

AROMATHERAPY LABOUR KIT

Using essential oils during labour has been shown to have a calming and beneficial effect on the mother-to-be. In a six-month study of essential oils used during labour at John Radcliffe Hospital, Oxford, two midwives found that some oils were particularly useful during birth. These included lavender (to reduce maternal anxiety and for pain relief), peppermint (to help stop nausea and vomiting) and clary sage (to increase contractions). Just under 600 women took part in this study, which concluded that lavender was the most favoured oil during labour. Many of the women giving birth said that lavender helped reduce anxiety and pain as well as lightening their mood. Most women preferred using a spray to disperse the essential oils.

It's worth familiarising yourself with any essential oils you intend to take into hospital, so you know in advance which work for you and which have little or no effect.

Clary sage
Can relieve pain and help with contractions; it is more useful on a compress than in massage.

Note: Clary sage is not recommended in conjunction with gas and air or general anaesthetic.

Geranium
Good for the circulation, and can help breathing during labour. Use to scent the delivery room.

Jasmine
Very helpful in childbirth as it helps to relax you and lift up your spirits during the particularly trying phases of labour. Good as a massage oil.

Lavender
Calms emotions, and relaxes you, helping to stop any panic you may be feeling. Can be used in a warm bath during the first stage of labour and in a burner or bowl of hot water in the delivery room.

Neroli
Good if you're feeling nervous or apprehensive about the birth. Helps you breathe slowly and calmly and focus on the task in hand. Put one or two drops on a handkerchief and inhale or use as a spray.

Peppermint
A drop on the forehead during labour can relieve nausea and vomiting.

Rose
In normal use, this is used for uterine disorders, as it has a toning effect on the uterus. Very useful in labour as it helps to calm

nerves and can help the circulation, encouraging deep breathing. Can be used in a massage oil during the second stage of labour, or as a bath oil in the first stage. Very expensive, though!

Labour Day

How do you know when you're about to begin labour? The signs that you are on the way to giving birth vary. There are, however, three things that can demonstrate your labour has begun or is about to begin.

Your waters break
Your baby has been protected by a sac of fluid (amniotic fluid). This sac will pop when the membranes surrounding the baby give way, producing a sudden rush of water, or, as is more likely, a slow, steady trickle. If you think your waters have broken, contact your hospital or midwife immediately, as there is a risk of infection to the baby. You will probably be immediately admitted to hospital. You must notify the doctor or midwife if the water is coloured; this may mean that the baby has emptied its bowels and is in distress.

A 'show' appears
When you are pregnant, your cervix is plugged with a seal of thick mucus. This can come away from your womb before your labour starts or during the first stage. It is actually a small amount of pinkish mucus, combined with a little blood. Don't rush off to hospital as soon as you see a show, as contractions may not start for another twenty-four hours.

Contractions begin
These often start out feeling like bad period pains. You will soon feel a rhythm to your contractions – they begin mildly, build to

a peak and then gradually go away. However, in the last few weeks before labour you might be experiencing Braxton Hicks contractions, which occur when the uterus is preparing itself for the real thing. This is also called 'false labour'. To determine whether it is real, either take a warm bath (if your waters haven't broken) or walk around a little. The false contractions will gradually decrease – whereas the real ones will continue! If your contractions become more intense and regular, you are probably in early labour. When they're coming every five minutes and you find you can't talk through them, it is probably time to contact your midwife or doctor.

THE THREE STAGES OF LABOUR
First stage

This is usually the longest part of labour. It begins when the muscles of the uterus are contracting, and continues until the cervix (neck of the womb) opens up or dilates to about 10cm (4") – big enough for your baby's head to pass through. This stage can last from six to fourteen hours, when the contractions have got going.

The first stage of labour progresses from the *latent phase* when you are contracting relatively mildly, to the *active phase* when your cervix starts to dilate, usually at the rate of 1cm an hour for first babies and 1.5cm for other babies. Contractions are usually between three to five minutes apart. Finally, the *transition phase* comes when your cervix has fully dilated from 7 or 8cm to 10cm. You will know when you've reached this phase because you may feel nauseous or actually vomit, feel hot and cold or find your legs begin to shake uncontrollably.

Second stage

This is the time from when your cervix is fully dilated to the birth of the baby and may take from one to two hours for first-time mums. You will now feel a strong desire to push and a pressure on your rectal passage. You will probably find it easier to push if you are either squatting, on all fours or standing, as opposed to lying on your back, as the force of gravity will help the contractions. At the end of this stage, the baby's head appears, and this is when your pushing should slow down to give your perineum more time to stretch, reducing the chances of you tearing. Your midwife will probably tell you how to push more gently, by blowing in short puffs to get through the contractions.

When the head has emerged, the midwife will check that the umbilical cord isn't around the baby's neck. All being well, the cord is clamped and cut and the baby's shoulders are delivered. The rest of the baby should slide out quite easily and you will then be able to hold your newborn child for the first time.

Third stage

This can take from five to thirty minutes. Now that the baby has been born, the diminished size of your uterus causes the placenta to separate from the uterine wall. Further contractions help to expel the placenta, and by gently pulling on the cord your doctor or midwife will then deliver it. Some hospitals inject a drug to make the uterus contract and deliver the placenta.

PAIN RELIEF

During labour, you may find you want some form of pain relief. If you do decide to opt for one of the hospital's drug pain relievers as opposed to using natural methods, don't feel guilty. Every woman's experience of birth is different, and if your body needs a stronger form of relief, you should take advantage of the modern benefits of having an epidural or an injection of pethidine.

Similarly, if your labour has to be induced or you need to have a Caesarean section, don't feel you haven't performed properly – there is simply no way of anticipating how your birth is going to be. Medical intervention such as the Caesarean operation can now save the lives of many babies and mothers who might have died a couple of decades ago.

What's on offer?
Find out which drug pain-killing methods are available at your hospital. During labour you should be able to choose your pain relief from the following.

Epidural: This is an anaesthetic which eases pain by cutting off any feeling from your waist downwards, while you remain conscious. It is particularly useful if you are having a painful 'backache labour', when the baby's head is pressing against your spine.

The epidural anaesthetic is injected between the vertebrae of your spine through a thin tube, which is left in place for top-ups. To receive the injection you have to curl up into a ball, with knees pulled up under your chin, making your back rounded. A drip is placed in your arm and you are monitored all the time, so movement is restricted. However, a new mobile epidural has been introduced in some hospitals, making it easier for you to adopt a comfortable birthing position.

You may have problems passing water with an epidural, and a small tube or catheter may be put into your bladder to assist you. Some women feel faint and have a headache after an epidural, while others get backache for some time afterwards. Your legs may also feel heavy for a few hours. If you do have an epidural, it is worth seeing a qualified osteopath a few weeks after the birth to ensure there has been no damage to the muscles around the spine.

Pethidine: This is a narcotic drug which could be given to you in the first stage of labour if you are tense and nervous and finding it hard to relax. It affects different women in a number of ways – you may feel relaxed and slightly drunk, or you might feel sick and sleepy. If pethidine is given too close to your baby's birth, it can give him or her breathing difficulties and cause sleepiness. Some doctors do not give pethidine for this reason.

The drug is usually given by injection in your buttock or thigh. It takes about twenty minutes to work and the effects last from two to three hours.

Gas and air (Entonox): This is a mixture of oxygen and nitrous oxide inhaled through a machine you can use yourself. It relieves your pain by making you feel high and can be useful later on in the first stage of labour. Some women find this has little or no effect, others feel light-headed or sick while breathing in. There are no harmful effects to the baby.

To take gas, you are given a hand-held mask attached to a cylinder. You inhale the gas through the mask, whenever you feel a contraction coming on. The gas takes fifteen to twenty seconds to work, so you need to breathe it in as soon as a contraction starts.

Drug-free pain relief

TENS (Transcutaneous electrical nerve stimulation): This lessens pain in some women and is thought to work by stimulating the body's own natural painkillers (endorphins). By using this method, you have complete control over your pain relief and are still mobile. TENS helps lessen pain for some women, particularly in the early stages of labour, while others say it has no effect at all. It has no effects on the baby. Four pads containing electrodes are stuck to your back where the nerves from your uterus join the spinal cord. These are connected by wires to a battery-powered stimulator, known as a pulsar, which can vary the intensity of the current. You hold the pulsar and control how much current passes through the wires to your back and, when your contractions get stronger, you can increase the strength of the current.

Ask if your hospital has TENS machines. If not, you may need to hire one a few weeks before your due date. It's worth practising with the machine before you give birth, just to get an idea of the sensation.

Acupuncture: This is an ancient Chinese practice which works on the principle that energy flows through many channels in the body. If this flow is blocked or unbalanced, a person becomes ill. There are about 800 different points along these lines which are thought to affect different areas of the body or internal organs. An acupuncturist establishes which points on the body need to be treated and then inserts fine needles into the affected areas to allow energy to flow freely again.

The idea of needles may put you off, but they only penetrate the top layers of your skin, so acupuncture is virtually pain-less. The use of needles is often reinforced with herbs and moxibustion – the warming of the skin by burning a herb, moxa, over certain areas of the body.

The use of acupuncture has been shown to be very helpful in treating morning sickness during the early stage of preg-nancy, and helping relieve pain during labour, or to turn a breech baby. It can also be used to induce labour by using needles in the legs, hands and sacrum. Acupuncture has been shown to facilitate an easier birth and even to help regulate labour; for example, if your contractions begin to wear off, the use of needles can re-establish them.

If you have decided to have acupuncture during your birth, the practitioner will usually begin when labour is established (at around the point when your cervix is dilated about 4cm). Pain relief in labour comes from using points between the thumb and forefinger, in the foot and above the ankle. Nausea can also be helped by using a point below the knee. Like TENS this works by stimulating your endorphins. Acupuncture won't have any adverse effects on you or your baby.

If you want to hire an acupuncturist to help you during labour, you should get to know one a few months before your due date. Not all acupuncturists are available for treatment during a birth – but it's worth asking!

Home Births

You may feel happier giving birth at home, rather than at hospital. The comfort and security of home surroundings make many women feel more relaxed during labour, rather than the impersonal rush of a hospital. Women planning a 'natural' childbirth may feel they are more likely to get the conditions they want at home, as hospital staff may want to intervene and use drugs for pain relief. A home birth also means you don't have to travel anywhere, nor do you have to move from one room to another as your labour progresses.

If you're set on the idea of a home birth, do discuss it with your doctor or midwife as early as possible into your pregnancy. If you're worried about safety, you should check on the availability of an emergency flying squad in your area so that, if a problem should arise, you can be taken to hospital immediately.

There are a number of reasons why your doctor may prefer you to have your baby in hospital:

* If you're having your first child, you are generally thought to be more at risk than someone having a second (if the first birth was uncomplicated). The first birth tends to be the longest and most unpredictable.

But more and more women are now choosing to have their first baby at home. Before deciding, bear in mind that no effective form of pain relief is available at home. This is a serious factor to consider.

* Women having a fifth baby are also thought to be more at risk.
* If you have any health problems such as diabetes, heart, kidney or circulatory disease or epilepsy.
* If you have had any problems during your pregnancy, such as anaemia or high blood pressure, your doctor will prefer you to have the baby in hospital. The same applies if your placenta is lying below the baby in your womb (placenta praevia), which can prevent the baby's head from engaging in the pelvis. This would mean you would need a Caesarean operation in hospital to deliver the baby (see Glossary).
* If your pregnancy continues for more than fourteen days after your due date, or if you have a premature labour at thirty-six weeks or less.
* If you are having two or more babies or if your baby is in the breech position.

How to have a home birth
If you are intending to have your baby at home, your midwife will leave you with a pack of sterile maternity equipment a few weeks before your due date. You also need to have made some of your own preparations. For a happy and comfortable home birth you need to establish a warm room with easy access to hot water, a loo and a telephone.

Home birth essentials
* Old sheets and towels
* Plastic sheeting for your bed, or wherever you decide to have the baby.

* Anglepoise lamp so midwife can see in an otherwise darkened room.
* Chair and/or floor cushions.
* Food and drink for those helping out!

Contact your midwife when labour begins – she will keep in touch to see how you are progressing. When your labour is well-established she will join you for the birth. The birth may be attended by your doctor as well, but the midwife is wholly responsible for your labour and delivery.

Birthing Positions

You may want to try a variety of positions during your labour, to see which suits you. Practising some of these in the last few weeks before your birth can help.

FIRST STAGE OF LABOUR
Standing
You may find that standing or walking about helps you during the first stage. Gravity helps the descent of the baby and can make the contractions less painful. Try leaning against your partner during the contractions. He can massage your lower back or just rock you gently.

Sitting forwards
Either sit upright on a chair, legs apart, and lean forwards or sit astride a chair leaning forwards onto a cushion. Sitting on the loo can be very comfortable, too.

Kneeling
Pile up some cushions on the floor and kneel down with your legs apart. Rest your arms and head on the cushions, or use a

large bean bag. Some women like to stay in this position for the whole of the first stage. If you are going to stay kneeling for long, put something soft under your knees.

Squatting
Squat, either using a small stool with the support of your partner, or by holding on to something in front of you. This opens your pelvis to its widest and helps your baby's descent.

All fours
Kneel down with hands and knees on the floor, slowly tilting your pelvis to and fro, without arching your back. When a contraction has passed, lean forwards and rest your head on your arms. This is a good position for backache labour where the baby's head presses on your spine because it is facing your abdomen, instead of away from it.

First stage tips
* Your breathing is very important. Focus on breathing slowly, evenly and deeply. At the beginning of a contraction breathe deeply through your nose and out of your mouth. When you feel the contraction is peaking, breathe in more shallowly, inhaling and exhaling through your mouth. Then return to the slower breaths.
* Take each contraction as it comes, rather than feeling overwhelmed by the fact there are many more to go.
* Staying upright will make your contractions stronger and more effective.
* Try to relax between the contractions, so you have the energy to face the next one.
* Grunt, groan, shout, sing or make any noises you want during labour – being noisy is a good way to ease the pain!

* Experiment with different positions to see what suits you. You might find your optimum position changes, depending on which stage you are at in the birth.

* Spending part of the first stage of birth in your bathtub can be very relaxing, especially in a long labour. If lying down doesn't feel right, try kneeling on all fours, filling the tub up completely with warm (not hot) water. Make sure your contractions have become established before you get in the bath, or you could slow down your labour. If you have a backache labour you could ask the midwife or your partner to shower your lower back while you're in this position.

SECOND STAGE OF LABOUR
Standing up
If this feels right, stand up and lean against your midwife or partner. During a contraction, keep your legs apart and push.

Squatting
If you have practised squatting before the birth, you'll find it easier to use this position during labour – holding on to either your partner (kneeling in front of you) or a stable object such as a chair. Another squatting method is to stand with your knees wide apart, held by one or two supporters. Or your supporters can kneel on either side of you, each one with a knee under your buttocks, giving you more support; put your arms around their shoulders and they can each place one arm around your back.

Kneeling
Two people can support you on either side, with your arms over their shoulders. Or you can try kneeling on all fours with your head and arms resting on cushions or a bean bag. This position opens up your pelvis.

Lying down

While this doesn't make good use of gravity, some women feel more comfortable lying on one side, with their body curled round and with their upper leg supported or being held back. This is better than lying on your back, as the perineum has more space to relax.

Tips for the second stage

* Don't feel embarrassed if you involuntarily open your bowels or leak from your bladder – the birth attendants will have seen this a thousand times before!
* Try to keep pushing steadily during your contractions.
* During a contraction, when you feel like pushing, breathe in deeply and hold it for a short period as you bear down. Between your pushes breathe slowly and calmly. Try to relax as the contraction goes.

Water Births

British women have been giving birth in water pools for almost a decade. When Michel Odent, a French doctor, began to offer women the use of pools at his hospital in Pithiviers, giving birth in water began to seem a good option. In the 1980s, several British companies began to offer portable pools for hire; since then, around 20,000 women each year have spent some time during their labour in water.

Many women find that lying in water during labour is very comforting and helps to ease the pain. It is thought that relaxation in warm water may help your uterus to contract more effectively as well as giving you more mobility. Being in a deep pool also means you are buoyant and can float and change your position easily. If you actually give birth in water, your baby will be lifted out as soon as it emerges, dried at once and then wrapped in a big towel, to prevent him or her from becoming cold.

If you have a water birth you will spend part or all of your labour in a small, deep pool of water at blood temperature. You can now give birth in a portable pool at home or in hospital and about eighty National Health Service hospitals now have water pools. However, following the death of a baby by drowning, many regional health authorities refuse to allow women actually to give birth in water. The Government position on water births is currently being reviewed.

If you would like a water birth, discuss it well in advance with your midwife and doctor, but you won't be allowed to labour in water if you have a medical problem during your pregnancy, such as high blood pressure, pre-eclampsia or diabetes.

If you're intent on having a water birth at home, you can buy or hire one of the selection of portable water birth tanks on the market (see Useful Addresses). These are usually about six feet (2m) in diameter and can hold up to three people!

——— 7 ———

The First Few Days

Just after your baby is born, you and your partner will be able to spend the first few precious hours alone with him or her. This is a unique and magical time, when you can begin to get to know your child. It is worth putting your baby to the breast soon after the birth as this is the best time for the baby to establish the 'latching on' reflex, and also ensures that he or she gets a few healthy mouthfuls of colostrum. After these special hours, your baby will fall asleep and will probably spend much of the next few days sleeping. You, on the other hand, may be on such a high that you lie awake thinking about the amazing events of the birth. This is quite natural, and you will be able to sleep later on.

Don't worry if you're not feeling entirely overjoyed by the experience – you may be feeling tired and dazed and not have the immediate rush of loving feelings that you had expected. Bonding won't necessarily take place as soon as you've given birth – it may take a little longer to fall in love with your baby. If you have had a difficult pregnancy or labour you may resent your baby, but these feelings will pass.

The first few days with your baby will be spent nurturing, caring for and getting to know him or her. You will also need to recover your strength from the birth so, if you've decided to return home early, it is essential to find someone else to do the shopping, washing, cooking and other household chores for you during the early days. Ideally, you will be returning home to a well-stocked freezer.

If you leave hospital before the baby is ten days' old or have had a home birth, a community midwife will visit you every day to make sure everything is going well and to help you care for the baby. She will also make sure you are in good physical shape, by checking your breasts, uterus and any stitches you have had.

Ten days after the birth, the midwife is replaced by the health visitor, a trained nurse who will care for the emotional and physical health of mother and baby. She won't come every day but will visit depending on how often you need to see her.

How Will You Feel?

Immediately after the birth you may experience some discomfort or pain as your body gradually returns to normal. But the joy of having a new baby usually minimises these problems.

If you had stitches because of a tear or an episiotomy (a cut to ease delivery – see Glossary) you may feel sensitive around your genital area, especially when you sit down, pass urine or stools. There are various natural ways to ease this discomfort:

* Use the homoeopathic cream Arnica or Hypercal ointment around the stitches.
* Take Arnica 30c three times a day for four days after the birth to help with any bruising.
* Each day, thoroughly mix two drops of lavender oil and one drop of camomile in a litre of ice-cold water, and sit in the water for a few minutes. Or use the mixture on a cold compress.
* Apply ice packs or bags of frozen peas.
* Bathe the area with a few drops of calendula tincture and lavender essential oil in warm water.
* Take the pressure off the stitches by sitting on an inflatable rubber ring.

Many women suffer from piles (or haemorrhoids) after giving birth. These are basically varicose veins of the rectum, caused by increased pressure of the growing uterus on all the veins of the pelvis. They can reveal themselves as small round lumps around your anal passage or may be internal. They may not be painful, or they may bleed, itch or burn. To ease the problem:

* Use a homoeopathic or herbal piles cream or ointment such as Hamamelis. Or take Hamamelis 6c.
* Try applying compresses soaked in witch hazel – you can buy this at a chemist.
* Increase the fibre in your diet to keep your bowels moving. Linseeds taken with water are an excellent remedy and ease the pain.
* Use two drops of geranium essential oil and one drop of cypress in a bowl of water and sit in it for as long as you can.

Breastfeeding

When your baby is born, your breasts secrete a substance called colostrum. This contains all the antibodies the baby needs to fight off disease and illness. It is richer in protein than your later milk and so helps the baby to sleep for long periods between feeds. Even if you don't intend to breastfeed for long, it's well worth passing on this vital elixir designed to nourish the newborn.

If your baby sucks properly on the colostrum, after a few days your milk-producing glands will be stimulated to produce a different kind of milk, called the fore milk, which looks thinner than colostrum. The fore milk, which your baby has at the start of every feed, is thirst-quenching and means your baby is getting a drink before the richer hind milk – the food part of the feed. This is followed on the third or fourth day by the richer mature breastmilk which is mainly made up of water with a solution of other ingredients, including fat, protein, sugar, vitamins and minerals. Breast milk contains the right balance of calcium, phosphorus and magnesium – all of which are important for growth and bone development.

Breastfeeding is good for mother and baby. Human milk contains essential fatty acids which can help physical and mental development. It also contains unique growth hormones and antibodies not found in formula feeds. A mother's milk is also good for a baby's brain and blood vessel growth, while protecting it from coughs, colds, chest and stomach infections. Breastfed babies are also unlikely to become constipated and their stools are soft – and not as smelly as those of bottle-fed babies. Feeding a baby with your own milk also means you don't have the hassle of preparing feeds, or washing and sterilising bottles.

While breastfeeding is the natural way to feed your baby, it may not come so naturally. You may find it painful and have to learn the correct way to position your baby on your breast. But don't be discouraged, you may just need advice on how to breastfeed properly. If you leave hospital soon after the birth, your midwife and health visitor will help you to find a comfortable way of feeding for you and your baby. And if you feel you need more support, you can get help from a breastfeeding counsellor – through either the La Leche League or the National Childbirth Trust (see Useful Addresses).

Basic breastfeeding tips

* Breastfeeding is like learning a new skill, so do ask your midwife for advice if it isn't going smoothly.
* Find a comfortable position for you and the baby. You might like to sit upright, supported by cushions, or lie down. Make sure your back is well-supported to avoid backache.
* Turn the baby towards you, with his or her head facing

your breast and nose lined up with your nipple. Give the baby support by placing your hand against his or her shoulders, not behind the head.

* Brush your baby's mouth gently against your nipple – his or her mouth will open. Draw the baby to your breast. You can tell if the baby is correctly positioned if there is more of your areola (the area immediately surrounding your nipple) showing above the baby's top lip than below the bottom. Your baby's gums should be working on the areola – not dragging on your nipple, which should be at the back of his or her mouth.

* Once the baby is at your breast you should feel a burst of milk – known as the 'let-down reflex'. When the baby has sucked on one breast for a while, offer the other one to prevent soreness.

* If feeding hurts or the baby doesn't seem to be getting enough milk, stop the feed. Don't pull the baby off – the jaws are clamped tight around the nipple. You can break the baby's suction by putting your little finger in the corner of his or her mouth (keep your little finger-nail short!). Then alter your position and start again.

BREAST PROBLEMS

Sore/cracked nipples: This is a common problem, especially if your baby sucks vigorously or is wrongly positioned at your breast. If sore nipples are not treated early enough, they can develop cracks. Solutions:

* You could try an aromatherapy massage. Using almond oil as a base, add 2–3 percent lavender essential oil with neroli. Roll your nipple between your finger and thumb as you massage, immediately after a feed. But do wash your breast thoroughly before the next feed!

* A good homoeopathic cure for sore, cracked nipples is bathing the nipples in an Arnica solution (ten drops of

tincture to 0.25l of cooled boiled water). For inflamed, tender nipples try using Chamomilla and for cracked nipples which cause smarting, burning pain, take Sulphur.

* Try using a cream – calendula or Rescue Remedy creams can be very helpful. Specially formulated nipple creams, such as Calendon, are excellent.
* Avoid using soap or bubble baths as these dry the skin, and try exposing your nipples to the air as much as possible.

Engorged breasts: New mothers will find that on the third or fourth day after delivery, when their milk comes through, their breasts are very swollen and uncomfortable, often feeling rock-hard. Solutions:

* Take some large, chilled green cabbage leaves, soften them with a rolling pin and place them inside your bra to cool down and soothe your breasts. This looks odd but is highly effective. Or place a cold compress, such as a flannel wrapped around some ice, against your breasts.
* Try taking a bath with two drops of lavender essential oil and two drops of geranium oil in the water. Soak a flannel in the water and hold this gently against your breasts. This should relieve some of the pressure. Gentle massage with a few drops of fennel essential oil in a light carrier oil (such as peach kernel) is also highly effective.
* Draw off some of your milk by expressing it by hand – simply massage the breast over a wash basin to encourage the milk to flow, or use a breast pump. There are different types of pump, so ask for advice before you choose one. You can buy a hand pump from a chemist, but if you want to use an electric pump – where you need to use little effort to empty your breasts – contact your local branch of the National Childbirth Trust or the La Leche League for hire details. These are excellent machines and well worth the small daily hire charge.

✱ If you are also feeling weepy and sensitive to the cold, many homoeopaths recommend taking Pulsatilla.

Too much milk: When your milk first arrives it may spurt everywhere – or the baby may take too much, become uncomfortable and cry. Solutions:
✱ Use a nipple shield to decrease the flow of milk.
✱ Use breast pads inside your bra to absorb any excess drips.
✱ Express a little milk before you feed, so the baby won't choke if it flows too fast.
✱ Don't worry – your milk flow will probably even out by the time your baby is eight weeks' old.

Too little milk: If your breasts don't provide the constant supply of milk the baby needs, try these solutions:
✱ Feed your baby frequently. Breastfeeding is a matter of supply and demand – the more your baby demands, the more you will eventually supply.
✱ Drink plenty of fluids. You need about two pints more each day than you usually drink.
✱ Stop drinking caffeinated drinks as these can reduce milk supply by overstimulating your nervous system.
✱ Drinking fennel tea is said to increase milk supply.
✱ Try using a compress with aromatherapy oils: one drop of fennel, one drop of geranium and one drop of clary sage.
✱ The homoeopathic remedy for loss of milk in the first instance is Agnus castus and, if this does not help you produce more milk, try Dulcamara.
✱ Relax! If you feel embarrassed about breastfeeding, find a quiet room where you and your baby can focus on the job in hand.
✱ Enjoy it! Make the most of this special time with your newborn. Most mothers will agree that it passes all too quickly.

Glossary

Alpha-fetoprotein (AFP) test – This blood test is optional and is usually carried out between the sixteenth and eighteenth weeks of your pregnancy. Your blood is analysed to determine the level of alpha-fetoprotein. Small amounts of this are produced by the baby and then pass into your bloodstream. If you have a higher or lower than average level, there's a possibility that your baby may be suffering from spina bifida or Down's syndrome. But there is only a *chance* that this might be the case and you will be given another blood test and further screening such as ultrasound or amniocentesis or the new triple test (see below).

Amniocentesis – This test is usually carried out between fourteen and eighteen weeks and can be used to check for abnormalities in your baby, such as Down's syndrome and spina bifida. First, an ultrasound scan is given to detect the position of your baby and the placenta. Then a hollow needle is inserted through the stomach wall into the womb. A sample of the amniotic fluid surrounding the baby is taken. This contains some of the baby's cells, which can then be tested for abnormality. Amniocentesis means a risk of miscarriage in about one woman in every 100.

Caesarean section – This operation is used when a woman can't have a vaginal delivery. The mother is put under a general or epidural anaesthesia and an incision is made in the abdominal wall and uterus. The baby is then removed. A woman might have a Caesarean for a number of reasons, such as: if her placenta is low down in the uterus, blocking her cervix; if the placenta has come away from the wall of the uterus; or if the baby is lying across the uterus instead of vertically, or is breech (feet first).

Episiotomy – This is a cut made in the perineum by a midwife or doctor, to enlarge the opening for the baby. A local anaesthetic is injected into your perineum, which is cut with very sharp scissors or a scalpel. An episiotomy is used if the baby is in distress and needs to have a rapid delivery or if your tissues are so tight that they hold the baby in or there's a risk of you tearing. On balance, it is preferable to have a controlled, pain-free cut than an uncontrolled, jagged tear, which could damage the anus.

Placenta – This is a membrane which is rooted to the lining of the womb, separating your circulation from that of the baby. It is formed when the embryo first settles into the womb lining. Oxygen and nutrients pass from your bloodstream, through the placenta and are carried to the baby along the umbilical cord. While antibodies, giving the baby resistance to infection, reach the baby in the same way, alcohol, nicotine, and drugs can also be taken to the baby via the placenta. The placenta also filters out the baby's waste.

Triple test – A new test for Down's Syndrome, this uses the AFP test result (see above) with levels of other blood chemicals to find out how likely an abnormality might be in the baby. Only available in some areas.

Ultrasound scan – This is a very exciting test in pregnancy, as it's the first time you and your partner can actually see an image of your baby. A layer of gel is rubbed onto your stomach and a transducer – a hand-held instrument – is gently moved across. This picks up sound waves from your baby which are then turned into an image on a screen.

Useful Addresses

Active Birth Movement
55 Dartmouth Park Road
London NW5 1SL
Tel: 0171-267 3006
Runs classes on active birth and yoga, and hires out birth pools

Folic Acid Helpline
Tel: 0181-994 9874
Monday–Friday, 2pm–10pm

Foresight
The Association for the Promotion of Preconceptual Care
28 The Paddock
Godalming
Surrey GU7 1XD
Send an sae for dietary and other preconceptual information

La Leche League of Great Britain
BM 3424, London WC1N 3XX
Tel: 0171-242 1278 (24-hour answerphone)

National Childbirth Trust (NCT)
Alexandra House
Oldham Terrace
London W3 6NH
Tel: 0181-992 8637

National Council for One-Parent Families
255 Kentish Town Road
London NW5 2LX
Tel: 0171-267 1361

Toxoplasmosis Trust
Room 26
61–71 Collier Street
London N1 9BE
Tel: 0171-713 0663

Accredited complementary medicine practitioners

Send an sae to any of the following for a list of registered practitioners in your area.

The British Acupuncture Association and Register
24 Alderney Street
London SW1 4EU
Tel: 0171-834 1012

The British Homoeopathic Association
27a Devonshire Street
London WIN 1RJ
Tel: 0171-935 2163

The International Federation of Aromatherapists
Stamford House
2/4 Chiswick High Road
London W4 1TH
Tel: 0181-742 2605

National Institute of Medical Herbalists
56 Longbrook Strec
Exeter EX4 6AH
Tel: 01392 426022

Suppliers of natural remedies

The following all offer a mail-order service.

Ainsworth Homoeopathic Pharmacy

38 New Cavendish Street
London W1M 7LH
Tel: 0171-935 5330

Aromatherapy Associates

68 Maltings Place
Bagleys Lane
London SW6 2BY
Tel: 0171-731 8129

Dr Edward Bach Centre

Mount Vernon
Wallingford
Oxon OX10 0PZ
Tel: 01491 834678

G Baldwin & Co

171–173 Walworth Road
London SE17 1RW
Tel: 0171-703 5550
Suppliers of herbs/essential oils

Splashdown Birth Pools

17 Wellington Terrace
Harrow-on-the-Hill
   Middlesex HA1 3ER
   Tel: 0181-422 9308
   Offers pools for hire

Further Reading

The Family Guide to Homoeopathy (Elm Tree Books, 1989) by Dr Andrew Lockie is an invaluable guide to homoeopathic treatments during and after pregnancy and for all the family. It contains many safe and simple homoeopathic remedies for a wide range of symptoms.

A useful book mentioning the various tests is *The New Pregnancy and Childbirth* by Sheila Kitzinger (Penguin, £9.99).

Liz Earle's *Quick Guide to Post-Natal Health* (Boxtree, 1995).

Index

A

Acupuncture 73-4
  during labour 73-4
AFP test 88
Alcohol 9-10, 15-16
  foetal alcohol syndrome
    (FAS) 16
Amniocentesis 88
Anaemia 38-9
Aromatherapy 28-9, 40-50
  labour kit 66-8

B

Back pain 39-41, 56
Birth, after the 81-7
Birth, preparation for 64-80
  what to take to hospital
    64-5
Birthing positions 76-9
Births at home 74-9
Birth, water 79-80
Breastfeeding 26, 62-3, 81,
  83-7
  breast problems 85-7
  preparation for 62-3

C

Caesarean section 71, 75, 88
Caffeine/caffeinated drinks
  23-4, 31, 47, 87
Calcium 22, 43-4, 47, 84
Common cold 41

Conception 8-9
Constipation 41-3
Contractions, Braxton Hicks
  58, 69
  see also Labour
Cramp 43-4, 60
Cystitis 44-5

D

Diet/dietary supplements
  10-14, 21-4, 27, 37-9, 42-3,
  46-7
  essential pregnancy diet
    21-3
  weight gain 37-8

E

Eclampsia/pre-eclampsia 24-5
Ectopic pregnancy 35
Embryo 19-20
Epidural 71
Episiotomy 82, 89
Exercise 7-8, 36, 40-1, 44-5,
  49-50, 52-6
  how to exercise safely 53
  simple exercises 54-6

F

Fatigue 45, 53
Fertility 9
Fish oil 24-6

Flower remedies 29-30, 65
    labour kit 65
Foetus 16, 20-1, 25-6, 36-7, 57
    and DHA
    (docosahaexaenoic acid)
        25-6
    final months 57
    foetal alcohol syndrome
        (FAS) 16
    middle months 36-7
Folic acid 13-14, 22, 39
Food
    see also Diet

G
Gas and air (Entonox) 72

H
Haemorrhoids (piles) 83
Hahnemann, Samuel 30
Herbalism 31-3, 38-50
Homoeopathy 30-1, 39-50
    labour and post-birth kit
        65-6

I
Illnesses/problems in
    pregnancy 20, 24-5, 28,
    30-1, 33-6, 38-51, 53, 58,
    60, 66-7, 73-5
    anaemia 38-9
    back pain 39-41
    common cold 41
    constipation 41-3

cramp 43-4, 60
cystitis 44-5
eclampsia/pre-eclampsia
    24-5
ectopic pregnancy 35
fatigue 45, 53
indigestion and heartburn
    46-7
insomnia 47
miscarriage 33-4, 53, 58
morning sickness/nausea
    20, 28, 30-1, 36, 48-9,
    66-7, 73-4
oedema 49
placenta praevia 34-5, 75
varicose veins 50-1, 60
Indigestion and heartburn
    46-7
Insomnia 47
Iron 22-4, 39, 42

L
Labour 66-74, 76-80
    pain relief during 70-4
    three stages of 69-70

M
Magnesium 43-4, 46-7
Massage 51, 59-61
    areas for massage 60-1
Minerals 22-4, 39, 42-4, 46-7,
    84
Miscarriage 33-4, 53, 58
Morning sickness/nausea 20,

28, 30-1, 36, 48-9, 66-7, 73-4

O
Odent, Michael 79
Oedema 49

P
Pethidine 72
Placenta 34-5, 70, 75, 89
Prematurity 25-6

R
Relaxation techniques 61-2

S
Smoking 9-10, 14-15
Stretch marks 26-8

T
Toxoplasmosis 16-18
Transcutaneous electrical
    nerve stimulation (TENS)
    72-4
Triple test 89

U
Ultrasound scan 89

V
Varicose veins 50-1, 60
Vitamins 22-3, 27, 39, 41, 43,
    49

Z
Zinc 14, 23-4, 27, 41